Uniportal/Single-Port Video-Assisted Thoracic Surgery

Editor

GAETANO ROCCO

THORACIC SURGERY CLINICS

www.thoracic.theclinics.com

Consulting Editor
M. BLAIR MARSHALL

November 2017 • Volume 27 • Number 4

ELSEVIER

1600 John F. Kennedy Boulevard • Suite 1800 • Philadelphia, Pennsylvania, 19103-2899

http://www.thoracic.theclinics.com

THORACIC SURGERY CLINICS Volume 27, Number 4
November 2017 ISSN 1547-4127, ISBN-13: 978-0-323-54903-5

Editor: John Vassallo (j.vassallo@elsevier.com)
Developmental Editor: Colleen Dietzler

Thoracic Surgery Clinics (ISSN 1547-4127) is published quarterly by Elsevier Inc., 360 Park Avenue South, New York, NY 10010-1710. Months of publication are February, May, August, and November. Business and editorial offices: 1600 John F. Kennedy Boulevard, Suite 1800, Philadelphia, PA 19103-2899. Periodicals postage paid at New York, NY, and additional mailing offices. Subscription prices are $359.00 per year (US individuals), $521.00 per year (US institutions), $100.00 per year (US Students), $439.00 per year (Canadian individuals), $674.00 per year (Canadian institutions), $225.00 per year (Canadian and international students), $470.00 per year (international individuals), and $674.00 per year (international institutions). Foreign air speed delivery is included in all Clinics' subscription prices. All prices are subject to change without notice. **POSTMASTER:** Send address changes to Thoracic Surgery Clinics, Elsevier Health Sciences Division, Subscription Customer Service, 3251 Riverport Lane, Maryland Heights, MO 63043. **Customer Service (orders, claims, online, change of address): Telephone: 1-800-654-2452 (U.S. and Canada); 314-447-8871 (outside U.S. and Canada). Fax: 314-447-8029. E-mail: journalscustomerservice-usa@elsevier.com (for print support); journalsonlinesupport-usa@elsevier.com (for online support).**

Reprints. For copies of 100 or more, of articles in this publication, please contact Commercial Rights Department, Elsevier Inc., 360 Park Avenue South, New York, NY 10010-1710. Tel: 212-633-3874; Fax: 212-633-3820; E-mail: reprints@elsevier.com.

Thoracic Surgery Clinics is covered in *MEDLINE/PubMed (Index Medicus)*, *EMBASE/Excerpta Medica*, *Science Citation Index Expanded (SciSearch®)*, *Journal Citation Reports/Science Edition,* and *Current Contents®/Clinical Medicine*.

Contributors

CONSULTING EDITOR

M. BLAIR MARSHALL, MD, FACS
Chief, Division of Thoracic Surgery, Associate
Professor, Department of Surgery,
Georgetown University Medical Center,
Georgetown University School of Medicine,
Washington, DC, USA

EDITOR

GAETANO ROCCO, MD, FRCSEd, FEBTS, FCCP
Director, Thoracic Department, Chief,
Division of Thoracic Surgery, Istituto Nazionale
Tumori, IRCCS, Fondazione "G. Pascale,"
Naples, Italy

AUTHORS

BENEDETTA BEDETTI, MD
Locum Consultant, Department of
Thoracic Surgery, Malteser Hospital, Bonn,
Germany

LUCA BERTOLACCINI, MD, PhD, FCCP
Department of Thoracic Surgery,
AUSL Romagna Teaching Hospital, Ravenna,
Italy

ALESSANDRO BRUNELLI, MD
Department of Thoracic Surgery, St James's
University Hospital, Leeds, United Kingdom

JIA-AN DING, MD
Department of General Thoracic Surgery,
Shanghai Pulmonary Hospital, Tongji
University School of Medicine, Shanghai,
China

SEKHNIAIDZE DMITRII, MD
Thoracic Surgery Department, Regional Clinic
Hospital, Tyumen, Russia

DIEGO GONZALEZ-RIVAS, MD, FECTS
Director, Uniportal VATS Training Program,
Department of Thoracic Surgery, Shanghai
Pulmonary Hospital, Tongji University School
of Medicine, Shanghai, China; Consultant,
Departments of Thoracic Surgery and Lung
Transplantation, Coruña University Hospital,
Coruña, Spain; Head, Minimally Invasive
Thoracic Surgery Unit (UCTMI), Coruña, Spain

KOOK NAM HAN, MD, PhD
Clinical Associate Professor, Department of
Thoracic and Cardiovascular Surgery, Korea
University Guro Hospital, Guro-gu, Seoul,
Republic of Korea

XUE-FEI HU, MD
Department of General Thoracic Surgery,
Shanghai Pulmonary Hospital, Tongji University
School of Medicine, Shanghai, China

MAHMOUD ISMAIL, MD
Department of Surgery, Competence Center
of Thoracic Surgery, Charité -
Universitätsmedizin Berlin, Berlin, Germany

GE-NING JIANG, MD
Department of General Thoracic Surgery, Shanghai Pulmonary Hospital, Tongji University School of Medicine, Shanghai, China

HYUN KOO KIM, MD, PhD
Professor, Department of Thoracic and Cardiovascular Surgery, Korea University Guro Hospital, Korea University, College of Medicine, Guro-gu, Seoul, Republic of Korea

RAINBOW W.H. LAU, MBChB, FRCS
Division of Cardiothoracic Surgery, Department of Surgery, The Chinese University of Hong Kong, Prince of Wales Hospital, Shatin, N.T., Hong Kong SAR, China

DANIA NACHIRA, MD
Department of General Thoracic Surgery, "A.Gemelli" University Hospital, Catholic University of Sacred Heart, Rome, Italy

CALVIN S.H. NG, MD, FRCS, FCCP
Division of Cardiothoracic Surgery, Department of Surgery, The Chinese University of Hong Kong, Prince of Wales Hospital, Shatin, N.T., Hong Kong SAR, China

ALESSANDRO PARDOLESI, MD
Department of Thoracic Surgery, AUSL Romagna Teaching Hospital, Ravenna, Italy

KONONETS PAVEL, MD, PhD
Surgical Oncology Department, Moscow City Cancer Hospital, Moscow, Russia

GAETANO ROCCO, MD, FRCS (Ed), FETCS, FCCP
Director, Thoracic Department, Chief, Division of Thoracic Surgery, Istituto Nazionale Tumori, IRCCS, Fondazione "G. Pascale," Naples, Italy

JENS C. RÜCKERT, MD
Department of Surgery, Competence Center of Thoracic Surgery, Charité - Universitätsmedizin Berlin, Berlin, Germany

MICHELE SALATI, MD
Division of Thoracic Surgery, Ospedali Riuniti Ancona, Ancona, Italy

ALBERTO SANDRI, MD
Department of Thoracic Surgery, European Institute of Oncology, Milan, Italy

MARCO SCARCI, MD, FRCS(Eng), FCCP
Consultant, Department of Thoracic Surgery, University College London Hospitals, London, United Kingdom

JOACHIM SCHMIDT, MD
Lead Consultant, Department of Thoracic Surgery, Malteser Hospital, Bonn, Germany

ALAN D.L. SIHOE, MBBChir, MA(Cantab), FRCSEd(CTh), FCSHK, FHKAM, FCCP
Clinical Associate Professor, Department of Surgery, The University of Hong Kong, Hong Kong; Chief of Thoracic Surgery, The University of Hong Kong Shenzhen Hospital, Shenzhen, China; Guest Professor, Department of Thoracic Surgery, Tongji University, Shanghai Pulmonary Hospital, Shanghai, China; Honorary Consultant, Cardiothoracic Surgery Unit, Queen Mary Hospital, Hong Kong

PIERGIORGIO SOLLI, MD, PhD
Department of Thoracic Surgery, AUSL Romagna Teaching Hospital, Ravenna, Italy

TAKASHI SUDA, MD
Division of Thoracic Surgery, Fujita Health University School of Medicine, Toyoake, Aichi, Japan

MARC SWIERZY, MD
Department of Surgery, Competence Center of Thoracic Surgery, Charité - Universitätsmedizin Berlin, Berlin, Germany

ZE-RUI ZHAO, MD
Division of Cardiothoracic Surgery, Department of Surgery, The Chinese University of Hong Kong, Prince of Wales Hospital, Shatin, N.T., Hong Kong SAR, China

HUI ZHENG, MD
Department of General Thoracic Surgery, Shanghai Pulmonary Hospital, Tongji University School of Medicine, Shanghai, China

YU-MING ZHU, MD
Department of General Thoracic Surgery, Shanghai Pulmonary Hospital, Tongji University School of Medicine, Shanghai, China

Contents

Nonintubated video-assisted thoracic surgery (VATS) strategies are gaining popularity. This article focuses on noninutbated VATS, and discusses advantages, indications, anesthetic techniques, and approaches to intraoperative crisis management. Advances in endoscopic, endovascular, and robotic techniques have expanded the range of surgical procedures that can be performed in a minimally invasive fashion. The nonintubated thoracoscopic approach has been adapted for use with major lung resections. The need for general anesthesia and endotracheal intubation has been reexamined, such that regional or epidural analgesia may be sufficient for cases in which lung collapse can be accomplished with spontaneous ventilation and an open hemithorax.

Several minimally invasive approaches for esophagectomy have been described, including robot-assisted esophagectomy and hybrid techniques, total transhiatal laparoscopic approach, esophagectomy using right thoracoscopy, combined laparoscopic and right thoracoscopic esophagectomy, and esophageal resection through mediastinoscopy. However, very few publications have focused on the uniportal video-assisted thoracic surgery (VATS) approach. The authors describe their technique of the minimally invasive esophagectomy using uniportal VATS as the thoracic step.

Interest in uniportal video-assisted thoracic surgery (VATS) is rapidly growing worldwide because it represents the surgical approach to the lung with the least-possible trauma. Specific training in this surgical approach is crucial due to its technical implications, to perform it safely while upholding the required therapeutic radicality. Novel strategies, such as interactive learning technologies, simulators, high-volume preceptorships, and targeted proctorships, play important roles in the training for uniportal VATS which, ideally, should be standardized, governed, and credentialed by national and international surgical societies to ensure patient safety and academic responsibility.

Fast-tracking patients in surgery has become standard in many hospitals. This allows for a shorter hospital stay and a complete organized pathway for treating patients. The operative trauma has an important role in the patient's recovery, as has the increasing use of minimally invasive procedures. In thoracic surgery, video-assisted thoracic surgery (VATS) procedures are aimed at reducing the operative trauma. One of the latest developments of VATS is represented by the uniportal approach, whose purpose is to reduce postoperative pain and morbidity. This article reviews the current literature and the authors' experience in combining uniportal VATS technique and fast-track surgery.

THORACIC SURGERY CLINICS

FORTHCOMING ISSUES

February 2018
Thoracic Surgery in the Special Care Patient
Sharon Ben-Or, *Editor*

May 2018
Fundamentals of Airway Surgery, Part I
Jean Deslauriers, Farid M. Shamji,
and Bill Nelems, *Editors*

August 2018
Fundamentals of Airway Surgery, Part II
Jean Deslauriers, Farid M. Shamji,
and Bill Nelems, *Editors*

RECENT ISSUES

August 2017
Quality in Thoracic Surgery
Felix G. Fernandez, *Editor*

May 2017
Disorders of the Chest Wall
Henning A. Gaissert, *Editor*

February 2017
Clinical Management of Chest Tubes
Pier Luigi Filosso, *Editor*

RELATED INTEREST

Surgical Clinics, August 2017 (Vol. 97, Issue 4)
Cardiothoracic Surgery
John H. Braxton, *Editor*
Available at: http://www.surgical.theclinics.com/

THE CLINICS ARE AVAILABLE ONLINE!
Access your subscription at:
www.theclinics.com

Preface

E Pluribus Unum (From the Many, Only One)

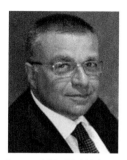

Gaetano Rocco, MD, FRCSEd, FEBTS, FCCP
Editor

Single-port or uniportal video-assisted thoracic surgery (VATS) is a surgical technique that in the past decade has evoked controversies that are still unresolved. The specific eye-hand coordination for the sagittal approach, the steep learning curve, the size of the incision, its location, and the mutual position of the instruments are all still debated among proselytes and opponents of this technique. Nevertheless, the popularity of this procedure is increasing, especially among Asian colleagues, who have widely adopted this technique since it respects like no other the corporeal and spiritual wholeness of the human body. Uniportal VATS has also contributed to differentiate generations of surgeons with the youngest ones being attracted by an approach that contains all the elements of minimal invasiveness with variations on a theme represented by the recently introduced subxyphoid and subcostal single incisions. However, the substrate of evidence that uniportal VATS is based on is far from solid. In fact, apart from retrospectively analyzed institutional or limited multicentric series, only a few randomized studies have been published, with controversial results. Nevertheless, the appeal of a 3-cm single incision to accomplish a major pulmonary resection on an awake or nonintubated patient, possibly without impinging on an intercostal bundle and using the most advanced refinements in technology for intrathoracic visualization, seems irresistible. This issue of the *Thoracic Surgery Clinics* attempts to provide an unbiased overall view of the uniportal VATS technique expressed by authorities in the thoracic surgical community. Indeed, this issue summarizes the technical details, the desired skill set, and the challenges of a unique approach among the many available in the thoracic surgical armamentarium: *e pluribus unum.*

Gaetano Rocco, MD, FRCSEd, FEBTS, FCCP
Thoracic Department
Division of Thoracic Surgery
Istituto Nazionale Tumori, IRCCS
Fondazione "G. Pascale"
Naples, Italy

E-mail address:
g.rocco@istitutotumori.na.it

Thorac Surg Clin 27 (2017) ix
http://dx.doi.org/10.1016/j.thorsurg.2017.08.001
1547-4127/17/© 2017 Published by Elsevier Inc.

The Geometric and Ergonomic Appeal of Uniportal Video-Assisted Thoracic Surgery

Luca Bertolaccini, MD, PhD[a],*,
Gaetano Rocco, MD, FRCS (Ed), FETCS[b],
Alessandro Pardolesi, MD[a], Piergiorgio Solli, MD, PhD[a]

KEYWORDS

- Lung cancer • Geometry • Ergonomics • Minimally invasive thoracic surgery
- Video-assisted thoracic surgery • Uniportal VATS

KEY POINTS

- The configuration of 3-port video-assisted thoracic surgery (VATS) is similar to a trapezoid, an unfavorable geometric shape for visualization with the standard 2-dimensional monitors.
- The uniportal VATS approach creates sagittal planes from a caudocranial perspective.
- The uniportal VATS approach preserves the depth and 3 dimensions of the intraoperative visualization.
- Uniportal VATS enables the operative surgeon to bring the operative fulcrum inside the chest.
- The uniportal VATS approach generates ergonomic advantages during the surgery.

INTRODUCTION

The idea of uniportal video-assisted thoracic surgery (VATS) was first proposed in 1924 by Singer, who devised an instrument to perform the surgical procedures through the same incision.[1] In early years of this century, Gaetano Rocco described the technique for the uniportal VATS wedge pulmonary resection.[2] From this report, the progressive refinements of this technique were associated with a broader range of surgical indications, including the major anatomic pulmonary resections for lung cancers.[3] Nevertheless, because of its relatively recent description and implementation, this approach had the potential and the relative urgency to expand the scientific

evidence about its benefits and to explore new areas of practice. Some articles have already demonstrated the advantage of the uniportal VATS in comparison to the traditional multiportal techniques in terms of the reduction of postoperative pain and hospital stay as well as a prompt return to daily life activities.[4] At the same time, there is a lack of great comparative or randomized studies aimed at verifying a consistent positive effect of the uniportal approach on the outcomes mentioned above, particularly in patients undergoing major lung resection for cancer. To this date, the geometric characteristics of uniportal VATS are known: one small incision without further dissection of the intercostal space with the

Disclosure Statement: The authors have nothing to disclose.
[a] Department of Thoracic Surgery, AUSL Romagna Teaching Hospital, Viale Vincenzo Randi 5, Ravenna 48121, Italy; [b] Division of Thoracic Surgery, Department of Thoracic Surgical and Medical Oncology, IRCCS Istituto Nazionale Tumori, IRCCS, Pascale Foundation, Via Mariano Semmola 81, Naples 80131, Italy
* Corresponding author.
E-mail address: luca.bertolaccini@gmail.com

thoracic.theclinics.com

simultaneous introduction of instruments in the thoracoscope through an ideal circular truncated cone, wide as a surgeon's fingerbreadth. The thoracoscope is handled to show the position of the instruments during the procedure with simple zooming in/out of the operative field. An enhanced hand-eye coordination to visualize and operate the thoracoscope-instruments ensemble is also required in uniportal VATS.[5] In this article, the geometric and ergonomic appeal of uniportal VATS is discussed to better understand the foundations of this approach.

A BRIEF HISTORICAL NOTE OF THE GEOMETRIC EVALUATIONS IN UNIPORTAL VIDEO-ASSISTED THORACIC SURGERY

In a comment to the first description of uniportal VATS lobectomy in 2011 written by Diego Gonzalez-Rivas,[6] it was suggested that the uniportal approach translates the thoracoscope 90° along a sagittal plane, bringing the operative tools to address the target lesion from a vertical and craniocaudal perspective. The uniportal approach was different from the classic 3-port settings, in which the lozenge configuration allows maximal convergence of the operative instruments from each side of the target lesion. The field of vision obtained with the uniportal VATS can be restricted by the short incision thoracotomy and the interference of instruments, but with the use of largely curved instruments and the 30° video thoracoscope does not present blind spots.[7] Nevertheless, the occasion for writing the first articles about geometry and uniportal VATS originated from the first world meeting on uniportal VATS held in Naples on 26 October 2012. At that time, some of the world VATS and uniportal VATS experts convened to assess the status quo and the future perspectives of uniportal VATS as a potential adjunct to the techniques in the thoracic surgical armamentarium (Fig. 1).[8]

GEOMETRIC APPROACH OF THE UNIPORTAL VIDEO-ASSISTED THORACIC SURGERY LOBECTOMY

Although uniportal VATS lobectomy is performed based on translational approach along sagittal projective planes, in the 3-port VATS procedure, the bidimensional geometric configuration of a lozenge produces interference with the optical source. The interference, in turn, creates in 2 dimensions a new optical plane with the genesis of a dihedral or torsion angle. Because, according to Euclid's elements, a plane is any flat, 2-

dimensional surface, the uniportal approach works along the camera motion to the target (view axis) and 2 planes (the VATS instruments).[7] Therefore, the geometric configuration of the uniportal VATS approach is entirely different from the standard 3-port VATS settings.[9]

Three-Port Video-Assisted Thoracic Surgery Lobectomy Approach

In the typical 3-port VATS lobectomy approach, small ports are used without rib spreading. The strategy for ports placement follows the famous baseball diamond configuration and corresponds to a trapezoid in plane geometry (Fig. 2).[10] The surgeon's eyes (ie, the 30° thoracoscope) are in point A; the target lesion lies in front at point B. The other 2 ports are placed at points C and D to allow for the placement of the left- and right-hand instruments and the triangulation toward the target in point B along 2 vectorial planes $(\overrightarrow{CB})$ and $(\overrightarrow{DB})$. The viewing axis is a vector $(\overrightarrow{AB})$; this is perpendicular to the operative port axis $\overrightarrow{CD}$ and follows the natural longitudinal axis of the patient (feet toward the head). Nevertheless, this setting fails to reproduce the real-life setting, where the surgeons and assistants position themselves around the operating table. In real contexts, many surgeons stand anterior to the patient in lateral decubitus; therefore, the real axis of the operation is translated posteriorly (Fig. 3). The posterior port (D) is translated along the viewing axis, and the surgeon is too far from the instrumentation. Also, if the assistant stands on the opposite side of the operating table, the visual axis would be completely different.

Anterior Three-Port Video-Assisted Thoracic Surgery Lobectomy Approach

The 3-port VATS port placement strategy has been modified, as described by Henrik Hansen and colleagues,[11] to cope with these technical and ergonomic issues, thus generating the posterior translation of the trapezoid (Fig. 4). The camera port (A) was brought more anterior up to the anterior axillary line (A'). The posterior port (D) was placed further caudally (D'). The utility port position (C) remains unchanged. Although the trapezoid was preserved, the axis $A'B$ was more comfortable for the operating surgeon.

Biportal Video-Assisted Thoracic Surgery Lobectomy Approach

After gaining experience with the 3-port VATS approach, Gaudet and D'Amico[12] realized that the posterior port (D') was not always essential,

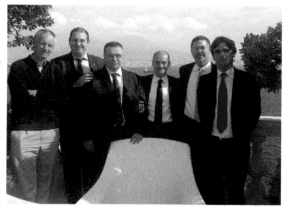

Fig. 1. Surgeons convened to the first world meeting on uniportal VATS in Naples (26 October 2012). From left to right: William Walker, Luca Bertolaccini, Gaetano Rocco, Alessandro Brunelli, John D. Mitchell, Diego Gonzalez-Rivas.

developing the technique of the biportal VATS technique (**Fig. 5**).

Uniportal Video-Assisted Thoracic Surgery Lobectomy Approach

Under general anesthesia and single-lung ventilation, the uniportal VATS anatomic resection usually starts by making a 3- to 5-cm access incision centered between the mid and anterior axillary lines in the fifth intercostal space. The incision is placed lower (fifth intercostal space) than the access incision used during multiple port cases (fourth intercostal space) to have a better entry angle for instruments and staplers and to achieve a better point of view on the hilum.

A wound protector is inserted into the incision. A 30°, 10-mm thoracoscope is placed at the posterior aspect of the wound and held in place by the assistant surgeon. This approach requires the translation of instruments 90° along a sagittal plane passing from point C, bringing the instruments to address the target lesion from a vertical, caudocranial perspective (**Fig. 6**). The approach to the target lesion is the approach that the surgeon would use in open surgery. The target lesion is in a projective plane with homogeneous coordinates and represents the point at infinity of this newly created cone-shaped parenchymal area.[13] The target is reached in a fashion similar to a coaxial approach: surgeons work with eyes and hands in the same plane (coaxial method), like

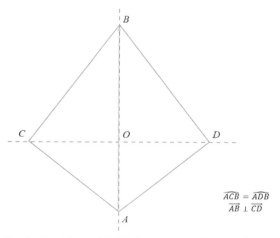

Fig. 2. Ideal 3-port VATS lobectomy settings. *A*, thoracoscope port; *B*, target lesion; *C* and *D*, operative ports. ($\overrightarrow{AB}$), axis of vision. (*From* Bertolaccini L, Viti A, Terzi A, et al. Geometric and ergonomic characteristics of the uniportal video-assisted thoracoscopic surgery (VATS) approach. Ann Cardiothorac Surg 2016;5:119; with permission.)

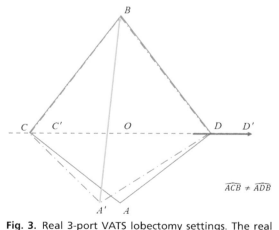

Fig. 3. Real 3-port VATS lobectomy settings. The real axis ($A'B$) of the operation is translated posteriorly. *A*, thoracoscope port; *B*, target lesion; *C* and *D*, operative ports. ($A'B$), axis of vision. (*From* Bertolaccini L, Viti A, Terzi A, et al. Geometric and ergonomic characteristics of the uniportal video-assisted thoracoscopic surgery (VATS) approach. Ann Cardiothorac Surg 2016;5:119; with permission.)

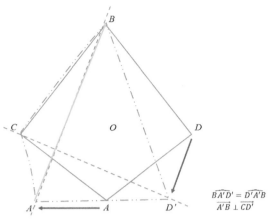

$$\widehat{BA'D'} = \widehat{D'A'B}$$
$$\overrightarrow{A'B} \perp \overrightarrow{CD'}$$

Fig. 4. Anterior 3-port VATS lobectomy settings. *A'*, thoracoscope port; *B*, target lesion; *C* and *D'*, operative ports. ($\overrightarrow{A'B}$), axis of vision. (*From* Bertolaccini L, Viti A, Terzi A, et al. Geometric and ergonomic characteristics of the uniportal video-assisted thoracoscopic surgery (VATS) approach. Ann Cardiothorac Surg 2016;5:120; with permission.)

open surgery but in contrast to 3-port VATS (paraaxial approach).[5] The optimal position of the camera and the instruments is decided in relation to the camera, depending on dissection at the anterior or posterior hilum. The monitor should be placed on a straight line between the operating surgeon, camera, and pulmonary hilum. The

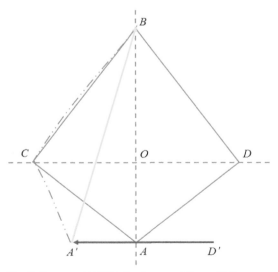

Fig. 5. Two-port VATS lobectomy settings. *A'*, thoracoscope port; *B*, target lesion; *C*, operative ports. ($\overrightarrow{A'B}$), axis of vision. (*From* Bertolaccini L, Viti A, Terzi A, et al. Geometric and ergonomic characteristics of the uniportal video-assisted thoracoscopic surgery (VATS) approach. Ann Cardiothorac Surg 2016;5:120; with permission.)

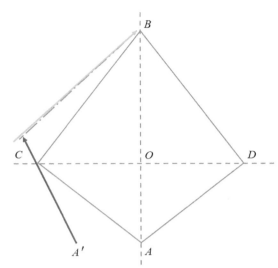

Fig. 6. Uniportal VATS settings. The thoracoscope instrument is translated to 90° along a sagittal plane passing through point *C*, bringing the operative tools to address the target lesion from a vertical, caudocranial perspective. (*From* Bertolaccini L, Viti A, Terzi A, et al. Geometric and ergonomic characteristics of the uniportal video-assisted thoracoscopic surgery (VATS) approach. Ann Cardiothorac Surg 2016;5:120; with permission.)

monitor should be ideally positioned to permit a moderate downward viewing angle of about 10°–30° without axial trunk rotation.[14] For the scrub nurse, the monitor is ideally placed just below eye level to allow a downward viewing direction of 0° to about 15°. Upward viewing angles, which may cause harmful neck extension, should be avoided. An axial rotation less than ~15° was considered ergonomically acceptable.[15] The angle of insertion of the camera can be adjusted to allow optimal circumferential visualization of the pulmonary hilum and the mediastinum. The uniportal setup requires maximal coordination between operating surgeon and first assistants. The operating surgeon can apply traction, expose, dissect, and divide the bronchopulmonary structures and the pulmonary vessels. The position of the camera and the instruments in a plane parallel to the intercostal space significantly reduces any torque forces commonly applied to the rib periosteum and the intercostal nerve bundle during 3-port thoracoscopy.[16]

MEDDLING OF INSTRUMENTS IN UNIPORTAL VIDEO-ASSISTED THORACIC SURGERY: GEOMETRY OF THE FULCRUM

To create a triangulation with largely curved surgical instruments, they should be crossed in the port access. The crossed instruments allow a better range of motion, but the resulting reversal of handedness significantly challenges the ability of mental adaptation by the surgeons.[17] One drawback of rigid instruments is that the incision acts like a fulcrum, limiting the movements of the device to 4° of freedom (**Fig. 7**). The fulcrum is the support about which a lever turns. Fulcrum, a word that means bedpost in Latin, derives from the verb *fulcire* (ie, to prop). When the word first appeared in the middle of the seventeenth century, *fulcrum* referred to the point on which a lever is supported (such as the oar of a boat).[18] The 4° of freedom make the instrument only maneuverable like an oar of a rowing boat. This effect makes it tough for the surgeon to, for instance, manipulate tissue or reach tissues from different directions without opting for another incision. The issue of addressing a target area from various directions, without adding to another incision, can be solved using curved or articulated instruments. The curved shape enables manipulation of tissues moving the shaft and rotating the tip toward the target. The tip motion is restricted to the degree of curvature of the instrument. If an action is required that needs a different angulation, another instrument should be inserted (**Fig. 8**). The curve motion is usually transmitted by rotating the entire shaft. In this way, not only the tip but also the curved part will turn, creating an unwanted hooking motion that can cause collisions with other instruments.

Conversely, the uniportal technique has the drawback of having the instruments and thoracoscope contending for the same space at the fulcrum of the port. The contention for the same space causes hand collisions externally and

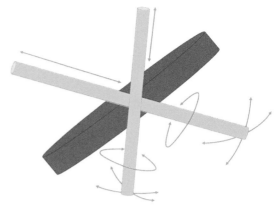

Fig. 8. Schematic representation of uniportal VATS instruments placing the uniportal access.

conflicts between the 2 instruments internally. According to previous laparoscopic evidence, there are 4 basic manipulation techniques for the instruments used in uniportal VATS. In vertical movements (**Fig. 9**), there is no conflict because both devices remain parallel with a broad range of freedom in the vertical direction. In frontal movements (**Fig. 10**), there is also no conflict because both instruments remain parallel to one another. The external crossing manipulation (**Fig. 11**) is required when the surgeon crosses the instruments by crossing the hands; the 2 instruments are passed externally, and this technique is recommended for holding to the left side of the monitor. In the internal crossing manipulation (**Fig. 12**), the surgeon passes the instruments of both hands internally, without crossing hands;

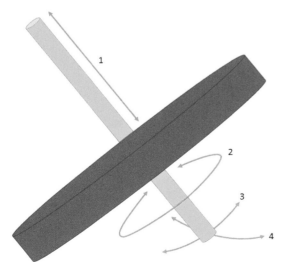

Fig. 7. Single-port access in the chest wall is limiting the movements of rigid thoracoscopic instruments to 4° of freedom.

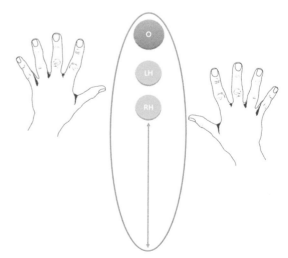

Fig. 9. The vertical manipulation does not cause a conflict of tools because both instruments remain parallel with a wide freedom degree in the vertical direction. LH, left hand; O, optic camera; RH, right hand.

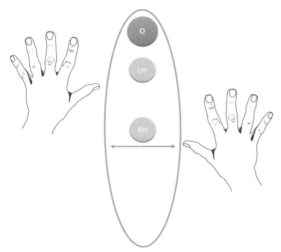

Fig. 10. The frontal manipulation does not result in a conflict of instruments because both remain parallel.

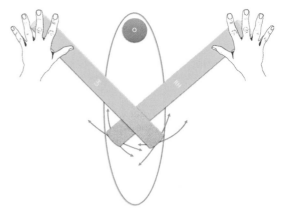

Fig. 12. In the internal crossing manipulation, the surgeon passes the instruments of the left hand over the toolkit of the right hand without crossing the hands and letting the instruments cross internally.

the limitations are the external hand collisions and the difficulty with tool tip manipulation. To avoid the internal conflict of instruments, a cross-handed approach using curved devices should be established. In the safe dissection of the target tissues, the surgeon's left hand must operate the instruments on the right and vice versa. These movements create a full degree of freedom in the fulcrum of the uniportal access; henceforward, there is no conflict of instruments, with a safe approach to the target tissue. If the instruments and thoracoscope interfere internally despite the performance of these movements, the problem can be overcome by putting the scope out to the port until the free motion of the instruments is obtained.[19]

ERGONOMIC CHARACTERISTICS OF UNIPORTAL VIDEO-ASSISTED THORACIC SURGERY
Ergonomics of the Assistant Surgeon

In uniportal VATS, the camera enters the patient's body from the incision; therefore, the thoracoscope should be placed as high as possible above the incision to provide enough space for instruments. The camera assistant controls the camera completely, and it is a challenge to ensure the quality of the image and keep the camera straight simultaneously. The camera assistant could use both hands to ensure the firmness of the camera. Fatigue caused by holding the camera for a long time reduces the attention of the assistant and increases the uncertainty of the surgery. A tip could be to fix the shank of the camera on the margin of the uniportal incision with a silicon loop to give the camera a fulcrum.[20] The assistant can use a single hand to hold the camera, decreasing the level of fatigue and helping to stay in focus. Single-hand camera holding can also provide an essential prerequisite for the sideways position. It was found that holding the camera contralaterally for a long time causes great discomfort. However, the ipsilateral camera holding takes up too much operating space and causes more collision of instruments and limbs, which reduces the comfort of the surgeon and fluency of the whole surgery. Holding the ipsilateral camera differently could improve the approach. On the upper and middle part of the thoracic cavity, the camera assistant could stand in the caudal region of the patient.

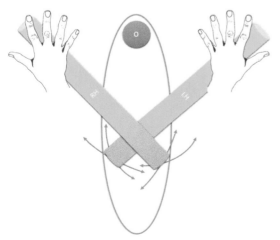

Fig. 11. In the external crossing manipulation, the surgeon crosses the tool of the left hand over the toolkit of the right side by passing both hands and letting the instruments cross externally.

On the bottom of the thoracic cavity, the camera assistant could stand in the rostral area of the patient on a proper footstool to keep the upper limbs 15 to 20 cm higher than the surgeon. During the entire procedure, the assistant should use the ipsilateral single-hand position as often as possible. This positioning gives more operating space, reduces the collision of instruments and limbs, and increases the degree of comfort and concentration. The fluency and accuracy of the surgery can also be guaranteed. In VATS, the camera lens is kept at a macroscopic distance in exploration, pulmonary lobe moving, instrument access, specimen withdraw, vessel or trachea cross, and tissue incision by the cut stapler, determination of the lobe or the segment plane, and observation of pulmonary ventilation in lung inflation, and so forth. The camera lens should be at a short distance in view of a small tumor, dealing with pleural adhesion, dissociating tissues such as vessels and lymph nodes, hemostasis, and suture, and so forth. To adjust the camera lens to a proper distance, the assistant should be well familiar with the surgical procedures, understand the intention and conducts of the surgeons, and be adaptable in any condition. The perspectives of observation commonly used in uniportal VATS are from anterior to posterior, from posterior to anterior, from top to bottom, and from bottom to top. The perspective from anterior to posterior is useful in the dissection of the anterior mediastinum and the front of pulmonary hilum; on the contrary from posterior to anterior is used in the dissection of the posterior mediastinum and the back of pulmonary hilum. The observations from top to bottom are useful for the dissection of the upper part of the hilum and from bottom to top for the release of pleural adhesions and the haemostasis of the thoracic wall.[20] At the same time, the adjustment of the camera angle also should be flexible. The camera assistant should stay focused when facing a long-time surgery with severe pleural adhesions, demanding separation of lymph nodes and vessels, and such. Also, an excellent camera assistant can expose the potential or undetected problems, helping to improve the safety of surgery.[20]

Ergonomics of the Operative Surgeon

The use of VATS entails some ergonomic problems, such as dealing with a large working area while assuming a rather static body position, eventually leading to fatigue of the legs, extreme movements of the upper limbs and the wrist, and, stiffness of the neck. The surgeon usually acts sideways from the patient during 3-port VATS because of the position of the trocars, which are apart from the endoscope. He should rotate his torso and lean over the patient to operate. This position causes a somewhat troublesome, unstable, and fatiguing body position, which should be maintained for the entire surgical procedure. During the surgical operation, the surgeon turns his neck and works in a different direction to view the monitor.[21] The self-reported physical demand after performing uniportal VATS was rated significantly lower than after conventional, 3-port VATS. It has been observed that the body posture during conventional VATS requires more elbow flexion (causing prolonged activation of the biceps) and more wrist flexion (causing greater fatigue) because the surgeon raises and abducts his shoulders, thus overloading the trapezius muscle.[5] Significant ergonomic benefits might be gained in the uniportal VATS environment because the viewing direction is brought back to the path orientation and restores the natural eye-hand target axis. The physical workload is significantly less challenging with uniportal than with 3-port VATS. The more neutral ergonomic posture during uniportal VATS may have resulted from manipulation without influencing instrument movements. Future research should evaluate the ergonomics in VATS major pulmonary resections, investigating the effect of ergonomic interventions on physical and mental workload.[5,15] Therefore, it is important that new instruments be produced with careful observance of the geometry behind the technique, the surgeon's needs, and the evidence-based acceptance for the use of these new tools in the surgical armamentarium.[22]

SUMMARY

Standard 3-port VATS has a geometric configuration of a trapezoid that interferes with the optical source with a creation of a new optical plane for the genesis of a dihedral or torsion angle not favorable with standard 2-dimensional monitors. On the contrary, the uniportal VATS approach of the lesion along sagittal planes from a caudocranial perspective realizes projective planes that preserve the depth of intraoperative visualization. The instruments, moving along this planes, enable the surgeon to bring the operative fulcrum inside the chest. Also, the uniportal VATS approach can improve the body posture during surgery because the surgeon can stand straight, facing the monitor, with minimal neck extension/rotation. The improved posture and more natural working direction generate an ergonomic advantage of uniportal VATS.

REFERENCES

1. Rocco G. Fact checking in the history of uniportal video-assisted thoracoscopic surgery. J Thorac Dis 2016;8:1849–50.
2. Rocco G, Martin-Ucar A, Passera E. Uniportal VATS wedge pulmonary resections. Ann Thorac Surg 2004;77:726–8.
3. Gonzalez-Rivas D, Paradela M, Fernandez R, et al. Uniportal video-assisted thoracoscopic lobectomy: two years of experience. Ann Thorac Surg 2013; 95:426–32.
4. Salati M, Rocco G. The uni-portal video-assisted thoracic surgery: achievements and potentials. J Thorac Dis 2014;6:22.
5. Bertolaccini L, Viti A, Terzi A, et al. Geometric and ergonomic characteristics of the uniportal video-assisted thoracoscopic surgery (VATS) approach. Ann Cardiothorac Surg 2016;5:118–22.
6. Gonzalez D, Paradela M, Garcia J, et al. Single-port video-assisted thoracoscopic lobectomy. Interact Cardiovasc Thorac Surg 2011;12:514–5.
7. Bertolaccini L, Rizzardi G, Terzi A. Single-port video-assisted thoracic surgery resection: the copernican revolution of a geometrical approach in thoracic surgery? Interact Cardiovasc Thorac Surg 2011;12(3): 516.
8. Bertolaccini L, Rocco G, Viti A, et al. Geometrical characteristics of uniportal VATS. J Thorac Dis 2013;5:S214–6.
9. Anile M, Diso D, Mantovani S, et al. Uniportal video assisted thoracoscopic lobectomy: going directly from open surgery to a single port approach. J Thorac Dis 2014;6:S641–3.
10. Sihoe AD. The evolution of minimally invasive thoracic surgery: implications for the practice of uniportal thoracoscopic surgery. J Thorac Dis 2014;6: S604–17.
11. Hansen HJ, Petersen RH, Christensen M. Video-assisted thoracoscopic surgery (VATS) lobectomy using a standardized anterior approach. Surg Endosc 2011;25:1263–9.
12. Gaudet MA, D'Amico TA. Thoracoscopic lobectomy for non-small cell lung cancer. Surg Oncol Clin N Am 2016;25(3):503–13.
13. Gonzalez-Rivas D, Fieira E, Delgado M, et al. Is uniportal thoracoscopic surgery a feasible approach for advanced stages of non-small cell lung cancer? J Thorac Dis 2014;6:641–8.
14. Hanna GB, Shimi SM, Cuschieri A. Task performance in endoscopic surgery is influenced by location of the image display. Ann Surg 1998;227:481–4.
15. Bertolaccini L, Viti A, Terzi A. Ergon-trial: ergonomic evaluation of single-port access versus three-port access video-assisted thoracic surgery. Surg Endosc 2015;29:2934–40.
16. French DG, Thompson C, Gilbert S. Transition from multiple port to single port video-assisted thoracoscopic anatomic pulmonary resection: early experience and comparison of perioperative outcomes. Ann Cardiothorac Surg 2016;5:92–9.
17. Arkenbout EA, Henselmans PWJ, Jelínek F, et al. A state of the art review and categorization of multi-branched instruments for NOTES and SILS. Surg Endosc 2015;29:1281–96.
18. Fulcrum. Available at: https://www.merriam-webster.com/dictionary/fulcrum. Accessed March 15, 2017.
19. Watanabe M, Murakami M, Kato T, et al. Rational manipulation of the standard laparoscopic instruments for single-incision laparoscopic right colectomy. Int Surg 2013;98:205–9.
20. Taotao G, Jie X, Runsen J, et al. "Ipsilateral, high, single-hand, sideways"—Ruijin rule for camera assistant in uniportal video-assisted thoracoscopic surgery. J Thorac Dis 2016;8:2952–5.
21. Young R, McElnay P, Leslie R, et al. Is uniport thoracoscopic surgery less painful than multiple port approaches? Interact Cardiovasc Thorac Surg 2015; 20:409–14.
22. Rocco R, Rocco G. Future study direction on single port (uniportal) VATS. J Thorac Dis 2016;8:32.

Management of Intraoperative Difficulties During Uniportal Video-Assisted Thoracoscopic Surgery

CrossMark

Marco Scarci, MD, FRCS(Eng), FCCP[a],*,
Diego Gonzalez-Rivas, MD[b], Joachim Schmidt, MD[c],
Benedetta Bedetti, MD[c]

KEYWORDS

- Intraoperative complications • Troubleshooting • Intraoperative bleeding • Uniportal VATS

KEY POINTS

- The more frequent and fearful complication during a uniportal video-assisted thoracoscopic surgery (VATS) anatomic resection is a vascular injury that causes a major bleeding.
- The incidence of major intraoperative complications during uniportal VATS lobectomy is low and, when they do occur, they are usually manageable.
- Emergency conversion to thoracotomy may be required; it depends on the experience of the surgeon and should not be considered as a failure.

 Video content accompanies this article at http://www.thoracic.theclinics.com/.

INTRODUCTION

Since the introduction of video-assisted thoracoscopic surgery (VATS) anatomic lung resection for lung cancer in the 1990s, this technique has experienced major technical developments and has demonstrated to be safe and effective for the treatment of both nononcologic (eg, pneumothoraces and malignant pleural effusions) and oncologic diseases.[1–3] Indeed, many authors have reported that the VATS technique is associated with decreased morbidity, pain, and duration of hospital stay and, regarding the oncologic procedures, it offers equivalence in terms of survival and recurrence rates when compared with thoracotomy.[4–6] These are the reasons why VATS lobectomy is now accepted as the standard surgical approach for early stage lung cancer and, in selected cases, even for more advanced disease. In the literature, multiple variants of the VATS technique are described according to port numbers, positions, and entry styles. For more than a decade, most surgeons performed VATS with 1 utility port plus 1 or 2 more assistant ports,[7]

Disclosure Statement: The authors have nothing to disclose. The authors certify that no funding has been received for the conduct of this study and/or preparation of this article.
[a] Department of Thoracic Surgery, University College London Hospitals, 15-18 Westmoreland Street, London W1G 8PH, UK; [b] Department of Thoracic Surgery, Coruña University Hospital and Minimally Invasive Thoracic Surgery Unit (UCTMI), Xubias 84, Coruña 15006, Spain; [c] Department of Thoracic Surgery, Malteser Hospital, Von-Hompesch-Strasse 1, Bonn 53123, Germany
* Corresponding author.
E-mail address: marco.scarci@nhs.net

Thorac Surg Clin 27 (2017) 339–346
http://dx.doi.org/10.1016/j.thorsurg.2017.06.002

thoracic.theclinics.com

until Rocco and colleagues[8] published the first case series of uniportal VATS pulmonary wedge resection in 2004. Since then, uniportal VATS has become an increasingly popular approach to manage most thoracic surgical diseases, owing to the potential advantages of reduced access trauma, less pain, and better cosmesis.[9]

Technological improvements like high-definition cameras, new specific instrumentation, curved tip appliers for vascular clips, and more angulated staplers have made this approach safer, widening the indications for single-port thoracoscopic resections.[10] Live surgery events and courses, together with a large number of videos posted on specialized websites, have contributed to accelerating the learning curve and the evolution of minimally invasive thoracic surgery. However, the learning curve of the uniportal VATS approach is linked to a larger rate of intraoperative complications, which often lead to an emergency conversion to thoracotomy. This article analyzes possible major intraoperative complications that can occur during a uniportal VATS procedure, and explains how to manage them effectively and safely.

MOST COMMON COMPLICATIONS IN UNIPORTAL VIDEO-ASSISTED THORACOSCOPIC SURGERY

The incidence of major intraoperative complications during uniportal VATS lobectomy is low and, when they do occur, they are usually manageable.[11]

The main complications that can occur during major uniportal VATS procedures and that may lead to thoracotomy are as follows.

1. Vascular injuries (more frequent)
   - Bleeding from the major vessels
   - Bleeding from the lung parenchyma
   - Other vascular injuries: subclavian vessels, superior vena cava
2. Airway injury
3. Technical problems
   - Fused or complex fissure, pleural symphysis
   - Emphysematous lung or absence of lung collapse
   - Difficult identification of the target lesion through digital palpation
   - Complex artery or vein, bronchus dissection, or a difficult anatomy
   - Calcified hilar and/or periarterial lymph nodes
   - Previous ipsilateral surgery
   - High doses of neoadjuvant chemoradiotherapy
   - Chest involvement

The more frequent and fearful complication during uniportal VATS anatomic resection is a vascular injury that causes major bleeding. The best strategy to manage bleeding in these situations is to prevent it from happening. Patient selection and an appropriate preoperative workup are essential to avoiding complications; in this setting, careful planning of the procedure should take in consideration:

- Patient characteristics;
- Size of the tumor;
- Position and radiographic appearance of the area of the lung to be resected; and
- Previous history of infections, which may increase the risk of an intraoperative bleeding (especially if dense adhesions are present).

The study and observation of the preoperative computed tomography scan is essential to identify vascular anomalies, hilar tumors, or calcified lymph nodes around the vessels, which require a more careful vascular dissection.

Vascular Injuries

The main causes of intraoperative bleeding in VATS surgery are the following.[12]

- Inexperience of the surgeon
- Difficult vascular dissection: fused artery or vein
- Calcified or malignant hilar lymph nodes stuck to the major vessels
- Vascular injury with cautery or energy devices
- Vascular laceration by the endostapler (limited angle or forced insertion) (Video 1)
- Vascular injury on the posterior wall with a right-angled clamp or scissors
- Failure of staplers
- Laceration during blunt dissection
- Metal or polymer vascular clip loosening or misplacement
- Excessive traction of fragile vessels (after chemotherapy, corticoid treatment, or in elderly patients)

Bleeding complications are frequent events during the initial phase of the VATS learning curve. Before approaching a VATS lobectomy, it is important to have performed at least 100 minor VATS procedures. In general, in centers with an established VATS program, at least 25 lobectomies should be performed annually by a dedicated surgical team (inclusive of nurses and anesthesiologists).[13] Team training is fundamental to deliver a safe uniportal procedure. Every member of the operating team should be aware of potential complications that can occur, and how they may be managed differently compared with thoracotomy.

Energy devices can facilitate difficult hilar dissection. Vascular clips on small pulmonary artery branches can be used keeping in mind the risk of inadvertent traction or accidental displacement of the clip during manipulation of the lobe.[14]

To properly control and repair bleeding, it is essential to have a high-definition thoracoscopic view as well as double articulated instruments specifically designed for VATS. One of the primary problems during bleeding is blood covering the tip of the scope, forcing the extraction and cleaning of the scope lens (Videos 1 and 2). It is important to quickly clean the lens without losing sight of the origin of the bleeding. Macia and colleagues[15] describe a method to clean the scope inside the chest cavity to provide better control of the bleeding site. It consists of using a small, butterfly-shaped, single-use lens cleaner (Endo-Clear) that is anchored to the parietal pleura during surgery to permit cleaning of the thoracoscope lens inside the chest cavity.

Ultimately, the decision for conversion is left to each surgeon's skills and patience. It is difficult to establish any set of guidelines for conversion to thoracotomy. However, our approach is straightforward: in the event of bleeding, a sponge stick is first applied on the injured vessel. Once the bleeding is controlled, a decision about whether or not to repair it thoracoscopically is made.[16] In case of a massive bleeding, an emergency thoracotomy to control the bleeding and avoid fatal blood loss is mandatory.

Type of bleeding

Minor bleeding Mild bleeding is usually not a troublesome problem and can typically be solved easily. A minor bleeding can be defined as a bleeding that originates from small vascular branches (generally smaller than 3–4 mm), small pulmonary tears in distal lobar arteries, or injuries created by traction or oozing from vascular stumps after the use of a stapler.[12] Minor bleeding normally can be easily controlled by applying pressure, vascular clips, or using energy devices, electrocoagulation, or sealants.[17] However, this kind of bleeding should not be underestimated, because it can represent a serious complication if inadequately managed.

Our first suggestion to control this kind of bleeding is to use metallic or polymer clips. Sometimes, excessive traction of the parenchyma while dissecting may cause small vascular tears that can be managed by releasing traction and applying compression.

A situation that needs to be particularly emphasized is the bleeding from the vascular stump after transecting the pulmonary vessels with an endostapler. Bleeding through the vascular stapler

line normally stops with compression but, if it persists, it can be controlled by using electrocoagulation or sealing materials. Special attention is needed to avoid melting the staple and causing additional injury to the vessels while using electocoagulation.[18] Occasionally, a reinforcing suture under the stapled line may be necessary (Video 3).

Minor bleeding is also common during lymphadenectomy owing to the small vascular branches afferent to the lymphatic system and can be controlled with energy devices or vascular clips.

Particular attention must be paid to bleeding originating from bronchial arteries in the deep subcarinal space, which are sometimes difficult to control. This is especially true when there is a retraction of an arterial stump, which can lead to the reason for conversion to a thoracotomy.

While performing paratracheal lymphadenectomy, extra care must be taken with the use of electocoagulation or energy devices in this area to avoid injury of the azygos vein or superior vena cava. For minor injuries, applying pressure can be enough to control the bleeding, but in case of major bleeding, the superior vena cava should be repaired by using a suture. This procedure should only be performed thoracoscopically by expert VATS surgeons; otherwise, an early conversion would be the best option to avoid catastrophic consequences.

Major bleeding Major bleeding is defined as a significant bleeding originating from the lobar arterial branches or on the main pulmonary artery or vein and can be life threatening if not properly managed. When this happens, Dunning and Walker[18] introduce their "swab-on-a stick" method to temporarily control the bleeding source. In fact, the bleeding produced by tear or traction while doing dissection normally stop after compression. Vascular injuries produced by accidental perforation with scissors, energy devices, or cautery normally do not stop with compression, and they need to be repaired openly or thoracoscopically.

Methods for bleeding control

Direct compression Direct compression on the vascular injury site is the first measure to be taken when bleeding occurs.

This is why a sponge stick already mounted on a long thoracoscopic forceps to enable compression in a reliable fashion should be readily available during a VATS procedure. Equally important is the use of the suction for blood removal and exposure of the bleeding site, preferably using a curved tip suction device (Video 4). An initial compression of 1 to 2 minutes is recommended. If the bleeding does not cease, a second compression of 2 to

3 minutes can be applied.[12] The use of suction is an alternative to the sponge stick in compressing the bleeding site. The suction creates a compression that stops the bleeding, and keeps the bleeding site clear of blood, not interfering with the suturing maneuver or the thoracoscopic view through a single-port approach (Video 5).

Use of sealants The use of topical sealants can be helpful in case of a small, controllable vascular tear. Sealants can be used even on minor oozing from the main pulmonary artery, which is a low-pressure vessel. On the market, there are several products available for topical use that accelerate the coagulation or stop the bleeding at a local level. There are 3 main groups of topical coagulants in relation to the mechanical action[19]:

- *Hemostatic agents*, classified into 4 groups according to their characteristics:
  1. Passive (or mechanical) agents (porcine gelatine—Gelfoam, bovine collagen—Ultrafoam, cellulose matrix—Surgicel, polysaccharide spheres—Arista) act through contact with bleeding sites and promotes platelet aggregation;
  2. Active agents (thrombin-based—thrombin) are biologically active agents, which participate directly at the coagulation cascade, stimulation fibrogen at the bleeding site to produce a clot. They provide hemostasis within 10 minutes and they are more effective in controlling bleeding than mechanical agents;
  3. Flowable (or liquid) agents (FloSeal, Surgiflo) combine passive and active agents into a single product and they act blocking the blood flow and actively converting fibrinogen into fibrin; and
  4. Fibrin sealants (Tissel, TachoSil) derive from human or animal blood products and imitate the final stages of the blood clotting cascade in the formation of a clot.

All hemostatic agents react with the blood in the surgical field, enhancing the blood clot and therefore requiring a degree of low-pressure bleeding, whether localized or diffuse. Some recent studies show the superior efficacy hemostatic matrix (FloSeal)[20] and of equine collagen patches coated with human fibrinogen and thrombin (TachoSil) over standard hemostatic material.[21]

- *Sealants*, composition:
  1. Fibrin (Tissel);
  2. Polyetiological (Coseal); and
  3. Mix of albumin and glutaraldehyde (Bioglue).

Sealants have a liquid appearance and many of them can be pulverized on the bleeding site. They require some time to dry and it is ideal that the area of application does not bleed at the time of use.

- *Adhesives*: the majority composed of cyanoacrylate (Hystoacryl, Dermabond) have a more restrictive use owing to its synthetic nature and rigidity. However, their high adhesive capacity allows them to stop hemorrhages from friable tissues producing moderate bleeding.

The efficacy of these hemostatic agents depends on the choice of the product for each indication and their correct application. Ultimately, the use of sealants should be reserved for situations where the defect is small or where the control by means of suture or ligation is complex.[22] Once the bleeding stops, further manipulation of the area near the field where the sealant has been applied should be avoided. If the bleeding persists, a direct suture should be applied.

Bleeding control through clips As described, the use of metal or polymer vascular clips is a safe option to divide small pulmonary vessels. The best option is to use 2 clips for the proximal end of small arteries and the energy devices to cut the distal end of the vessel. In this way, accidental displacement of the distal clips while manipulating the lobe can be avoided, and inclusion of the clip in the stapler line when dividing the fissure can be prevented. Sealing the vessel at the distal end is an additional safety measure to prevent the proximal stump from bleeding in the event of a displaced proximal clip.[23]

If an accidental proximal clip displacement occurs during surgical manipulation, it is usually still possible to apply a new clip if there is sufficient length to secure it at the base of the vessel. It has to be kept in mind that misplacement of the clip could cause irreversible damage to the pulmonary artery. Bleeding at the distal stump as a consequence of manipulation may sometimes cease with direct coagulation, using energy devices, or, in some circumstances, by suturing the stump.

Bleeding control through a direct suture Major bleeding that cannot be controlled otherwise must be repaired through a direct suture. Performing a direct suture repair on the pulmonary artery or vein during a VATS procedure is very challenging and should only be performed by expert VATS surgeons. The first measure must always be to compress the bleeding site and maintain a calm approach to the situation.

In the literature, many methods of suturing the main pulmonary vessels are described. Liu and colleagues[24] described a suction-compression angiorrhaphy technique to overcome serious bleeding from a vascular injury during VATS. They describe the control of the bleeding with an initial phase of compression (with endoscopic suction) and then the performance of an angiorrhaphy with suture. The vascular suture repair is performed using Prolene 5-0 and it can be implemented in 1 of 3 ways depending on the size of the defect and its location.

1. Defects of less than 5 mm: a direct suture repair is performed while providing compression.
2. Defects of greater than 5 mm (but not exceeding one-third of the size of the vessel circumference): an Allis clamp is used to initially close the defect orifice, and then a direct suture repair of the defect is performed.
3. Defects that exceed one-third of the size of the vessel circumference: an Allis clamp is used to initially close the defect orifice and then an atraumatic clamp is used to clamp the proximal end of the artery. The Allis clamp is then removed and a suture repair of the defect is performed.

Other authors have described preventive control techniques and pulmonary artery clamping during VATS dissection in complex cases such as proximal hilar tumors or calcified adenopathies involving arteries. In these circumstances, they recommend a correct proximal and distal mobilization for good vascular control.[25] Watanabe and colleagues[26] introduced the technique of preventive pulmonary artery clamping using 1-0 silk suture. The authors describe the clamping of the main pulmonary artery through the placement of a double 1-0 silk suture. This process is a good precaution for expected bleeding; however, this procedure is not recommended to be performed on every patient, because the suture clamp technique might cause injury on the intima of the pulmonary artery because of excessive clamping force. Another method is to use an atraumatic instrument like a ring forceps to grasp the artery and stop the bleeding as a first step, and then perform a thoracoscopic suture repair (Video 6). This allows us to better assess the defect and apply the suture with more precision and safety. Bleeding originating from a vascular stump, which does not stop after compression, must be repaired with a suture below the stapler line, preferably using a 40 or 5-0 Prolene. To repair the defect through a uniportal approach, bimanual instrumentation is crucial, keeping the camera in a posterior position and the instruments at the anterior position; the thoracoscopic curved suction is kept in the left hand (to effect compression and clearance of the bleeding site) and the needle holder is in the right hand. Owing to the fragility of the pulmonary artery, extra care must be taken with the traction of the sutures, especially when tying the knots. In the event of frail injured vessels or a significant laceration on the base of the pulmonary artery, reinforcement of the suture with Teflon patches is recommended.

Tips and tricks in case of bleeding

General Tips
- Follow the algorithm as in **Fig. 1**.
- The best way to avoid intraoperative events is to prevent them.
  - Adequate preoperative preparation of the patient.
  - Assess the anatomy from the preoperative computed tomography scan.
  - An instrument or stapler should never be forced, because resistance normally indicates important tissue in the way.
  - A leader can be used when introducing the stapler if the angle of the vessel is not optimal.
  - Beware of silk .suture cutting through the pulmonary artery
  - Good visualization of the vascular structures should be achieved throughout the procedure.
  - For improved safety, entry and exit point near the vessels should be cleared from lymph nodes.
- Always keep a sponge on a stick on the back table.
- Have always a plan B or alternative strategy in planning the procedure.
- Beware of anatomic variations.
- If serious bleeding occurs, the surgeon should initially apply pressure, release tension on the lobe, and acquire adequate backup, if needed. Once the injury can be assessed, the decision to repair or convert to open thoracotomy should be made. Conversion can be done through a natural extension of the incision or a standard posterolateral thoracotomy. In difficult cases, it is often best to initially obtain control of the main pulmonary artery with a tape or vessel loop such that a tourniquet can be applied for repair and control when needed.

Endoscopic Stapling
- Prevent complications by releasing tension on the vessel when stapling.

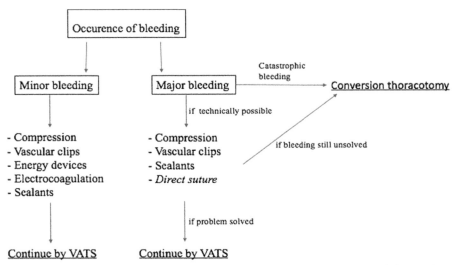

Fig. 1. Algorithm for the management of intraoperative bleeding. VATS, video-assisted thoracoscopic surgery.

- Encircle the main pulmonary artery every time that there are concerns about arterial dissection.
- Beware of erosion of lymph nodes in the vessels.
- Do not continue to dissect when there is bleeding and there is not good visualization: apply pressure on the point of bleeding and continue the dissection in another region.

Bleeding from the pulmonary artery
- Biggest fear in VATS surgery; maintaining a calm approach is beneficial for the operating surgeon and his or her team.
- Most bleeders stop applying some pressure with a sponge stick.
- Release retraction immediately.
- Use sealing material, if needed.

Bleeding from the pulmonary vein
- It normally stops with compression and time.
- If not, sealing materials or suturing are options.
- Do not convert too soon, because the bleeding usually stops and the operation can be finished by VATS.

Bleeding from the lung parenchyma
- Generally, in patients with adhesions or by redo operations.
- As a rule, this bleeding stops without big interventions.

Airway Injuries

Injuries of the airways are a rare complication and, normally, they represent a cause of conversion to thoracotomy to repair the damage. Here is a list of the possible causes of an airway injury

- Failure of the stapler leading to a massive air leak on a patient with severe emphysema or a fused fissure;
- Bronchus or trachea injury by the endotracheal tube; and
- Transection of the bronchus for another lobe during a lobectomy while completing the fissure (for example transection of the middle lobe bronchus during a right upper lobectomy).[27]

Technical Problems

Many technical problems can lead to intraoperative complications and, therefore, to conversion.

- A *fused or complex fissure or true pleural symphysis* presents a technical challenge to VATS lobectomy. To perform an adequate adhesiolysis, it is important to find the correct plane between the tissues and to create a space using a combination of sharp and blunt dissection. In case of fused fissure, we advocate a fissure-less technique, that is, by leaving the fissure to be divided last. Especially in case of lower lobectomies, with the uniportal approach, is possible to create a tunnel following the bifurcation of the veins and the bronchi up to the surface of the pulmonary artery. At that point, is easy to slide the anvil of the stapler into the fissure and divide it open (Video 7).
- An *emphysematous lung or the absence of lung collapse* can cause a difficult intraoperative situation owing to the small operative space. We recommend adequate muscle

relaxation to drop the diaphragm as much as possible and to apply suction through the double-lumen tube. Compression of the emphysematous lung also helps with deflation. The surgeon must be patient at the beginning of the operation to set up the best conditions to progress later. Rushing through the initial part of the surgery will cost more time and hassle later.

- The *difficult identification of the target lesion through digital palpation* (mostly, small nodules) is often a reason for conversion. However, new techniques to localize nodules are now available in larger centers.
- *Complex artery or vein, or bronchus dissection, or a difficult anatomy* can also be a critical point, although with improving surgeon experience and familiarity with VATS lobectomy these cases can be accomplished.
- The presence of *calcified hilar and/or periarterial lymph nodes* can complicate vascular dissection: the key in these cases is to find the adventitial plane.[14] Then, through bimanual instrumentation, the dissection can be performed with simple instruments (curved forceps, long scissors, suction and a conventional dissector); in really complex situations is possible to staple 2 anatomic structures together as described by Kohno and colleagues.[28]
- A *previous ipsilateral surgery* is also no longer a contraindication, because good outcomes of redo VATS surgery have been reported.[29]
- The uses of *high doses of neoadjuvant chemoradiotherapy* have previously been considered a relative contraindication, but VATS lobectomy can be performed safely and effectively in these patients.[30] Although surgery is technically challenging, isolating the main pulmonary artery within the pericardium allows an easy way to gain proximal control.
- *Chest involvement* requires thoracotomy for resection, but VATS can be used to perform the lobectomy and allow placement of the better incision to the chest wall removal. Recently, dedicated instruments have been developed to facilitate a through VATS approach to chest wall resection. The main issue to consider is whether the defect needs repair with a patch to avoid lung herniation.

CONVERSION TO THORACOTOMY

According to the literature, the conversion rate to thoracotomy is around 4%.[31,32] The conversion to open surgery should never be considered as a failure of VATS, but rather as a last line of defense to guarantee the patient's safety. It is fundamental to know when the surgery should be converted, and this depends on the experience of each surgeon. Even though, in expert hands, the great majority of vascular lesions can be controlled by VATS, there are situations, such as significant tears in the main pulmonary artery, when a prompt conversion to thoracotomy is required. It is important to always keep compression of the bleeding site and maintain an acceptable thoracoscopic view while converting to avoid catastrophic bleeding.[33]

SUMMARY

VATS procedures for anatomic resections are beneficial to patients. Intraoperative complications are rare and can be resolved thoracoscopically in the majority of cases. Appropriate knowledge of the anatomy and preoperative planning are essential in avoiding problems. Bleeding is the most common and feared complication while performing a VATS lobectomy but, for experienced VATS surgeons, there are many techniques to manage the bleeding thoracoscopically. If there is any concern or a major bleeding occurs, the conversion to emergency thoracotomy should be performed promptly, especially at the beginning of the VATS lobectomy learning curve.

SUPPLEMENTARY DATA

Supplementary data related to this article can be found online at 10.1016/j.thorsurg.2017.06.002.

REFERENCES

1. Van Schil PE. Treatment of pneumothorax: minimally or maximally invasive? Eur J Cardiothorac Surg 2016;49(3):868–9.
2. Landreneau RJ, Hazelrigg SR, Ferson PF, et al. Thoracoscopic resection of 85 pulmonary lesions. Ann Thorac Surg 1992;54:415–9 [discussion: 419–20].
3. Swanson SJ, Herndon JE 2nd, D'Amico TA, et al. Video-assisted thoracic surgery lobectomy: report of CALGB 39802–a prospective, multiinstitution feasibility study. J Clin Oncol 2007;25:4993–7.
4. Paul S, Altorki NK, Sheng S, et al. Thoracoscopic lobectomy is associated with lower morbidity than open lobectomy: a propensity-matched analysis from the STS database. J Thorac Cardiovasc Surg 2010;139:366–78.
5. Paul S, Sedrakyan A, Chiu YL, et al. Outcomes after lobectomy using thoracoscopy vs thoracotomy: a comparative effectiveness analysis utilizing the Nationwide Inpatient Sample database. Eur J Cardiothorac Surg 2013;43:813–7.

6. Jeon JH, Kang CH, Kim HS, et al. Video-assisted thoracoscopic lobectomy in non-small-cell lung cancer patients with chronic obstructive pulmonary disease is associated with lower pulmonary complications than open lobectomy: a propensity score-matched analysis. Eur J Cardiothorac Surg 2014;45:640–5.

7. McKenna RJ Jr, Houck W, Fuller CB. Video-assisted thoracic surgery lobectomy: experience with 1,100 cases. Ann Thorac Surg 2006;81:421–5 [discussion: 425–6].

8. Rocco G, Martin-Ucar A, Passera E. Uniportal VATS wedge pulmonary resections. Ann Thorac Surg 2004;77:726–8.

9. Jutley RS, Khalil MW, Rocco G. Uniportal vs standard three-port VATS technique for spontaneous pneumothorax: comparison of post-operative pain and residual paraesthesia. Eur J Cardiothorac Surg 2005;28:43–6.

10. Gonzalez-Rivas D. Recent advances in uniportal video-assisted thoracoscopic surgery. Chin J Cancer Res 2015;27(1):90–3.

11. Flores RM, Ihekweazu U, Dycoco J, et al. Video-assisted thoracoscopic surgery (VATS) lobectomy: catastrophic intraoperative complications. J Thorac Cardiovasc Surg 2011;142(6):1412–7.

12. Gonzalez-Rivas D, Stupnik T, Fernandez R, et al. Intraoperative bleeding control by uniportal video-assisted thoracoscopic surgery. Eur J Cardiothorac Surg 2016;49(Suppl 1):i17–24.

13. McKenna R. Complications and learning curves for video-assisted thoracic surgery lobectomy. Thorac Surg Clin 2008;18:275–80.

14. Fernández Prado R, Fieira Costa E, Delgado Roel M, et al. Management of complications by uniportal video-assisted thoracoscopic surgery. J Thorac Dis 2014;6(S6):S669–73.

15. Macia I, Gossot D. Maintaining a clear vision during long-lasting thoracoscopic procedures. Interact Cardiovasc Thorac Surg 2010;11:522–4.

16. Hanna JM, Berry MF, D'Amico TA. Contraindications of video-assisted thoracoscopic surgical lobectomy and determinants of conversion to open. J Thorac Dis 2013;5(S3):S182–9.

17. Demmy TL, James TA, Swanson SJ, et al. Troubleshooting video-assisted thoracic surgery lobectomy. Ann Thorac Surg 2005;79:1744–52 [discussion: 1753].

18. Dunning J, Walker WS. Pulmonary artery bleeding caused during VATS lobectomy. Ann Cardiothorac Surg 2012;1:109–10.

19. Spotnitz WD. Hemostats, sealants, and adhesives: a practical guide for the surgeon. Am Surg 2012;78:1305–21.

20. D'Andrilli A, Cavaliere I, Maurizi G, et al. Evaluation of the efficacy of a haemostatic matrix for control of intraoperative and postoperative bleeding in major lung surgery: a prospective randomized study. Eur J Cardiothorac Surg 2014;48(5):679–83.

21. Maisano F, Kjaergård HK, Bauernschmitt R, et al. TachoSil surgical patch versus conventional haemostatic fleece material for control of bleeding in cardiovascular surgery: a randomised controlled trial. Eur J Cardiothorac Surg 2009;36:708–14.

22. Forcillo J, Perrault LP. Armentarium of topical hemostatic products in cardiovascular surgery: an update. Transfus Apher Sci 2014;50:26–31.

23. Igai H, Kamiyoshihara M, Ibe T, et al. Troubleshooting for bleeding in thoracoscopic anatomic pulmonary resection. Asian Cardiovasc Thorac Ann 2017;25(1):35–40.

24. Xiao ZL, Mei JD, Pu Q, et al. Technical strategy for dealing with bleeding during thoracoscopic lung surgery. Ann Cardiothorac Surg 2014;3(2):213–5.

25. Nakanishi R, Oka S, Odate S. Video-assisted thoracic surgery major pulmonary resection requiring control of the main pulmonary artery. Interact Cardiovasc Thorac Surg 2009;9:618–22.

26. Watanabe A, Koyanagi T, Nakashima S, et al. How to clamp the main pulmonary artery during video-assisted thoracoscopic surgery lobectomy. Eur J Cardiothorac Surg 2007;31:129–31.

27. Samson P, Guitron J, Reed MF, et al. Predictors of conversion to thoracotomy for video-assisted thoracoscopic lobectomy: a retrospective analysis and the influence of computed tomography-based calcification assessment. J Thorac Cardiovasc Surg 2013;145:1512–8.

28. Kohno T, Fujimori S, Kishi K, et al. Safe and effective minimally invasive approaches for small ground glass opacity. Ann Thorac Surg 2010;89(6):S2114–7.

29. Akiba T, Marushima H, Kobayashi S, et al. Video-assisted thoracic surgery for recurrent primary spontaneous pneumothorax in reoperated chests. Surg Today 2009;39(11):944–6.

30. Petersen RP, Pham D, Toloza EM, et al. Thoracoscopic lobectomy: a safe and effective strategy for patients receiving induction therapy for non-small cell lung cancer. Ann Thorac Surg 2006;82:214–8 [discussion: 219].

31. Yamashita S, Tokuishi K, Moroga T, et al. Totally thoracoscopic surgery and troubleshooting for bleeding in nonsmall cell lung cancer. Ann Thorac Surg 2013;95:994–9.

32. Mei J, Pu Q, Liao H, et al. A novel method for troubleshooting vascular injury during anatomic thoracoscopic pulmonary resection without conversion to thoracotomy. Surg Endosc 2013;27:530–7.

33. Kamiyoshihara M, Nagashima T, Ibe T, et al. A tip for controlling the main pulmonary artery during video-assisted thoracic major pulmonary resection: the outside-field vascular clamping technique. Interact Cardiovasc Thorac Surg 2010;11(5):693–5.

Hybrid Theater and Uniportal Video-Assisted Thoracic Surgery
The Perfect Match for Lung Nodule Localization

Ze-Rui Zhao, MD, Rainbow W.H. Lau, MBChB, FRCS, Calvin S.H. Ng, MD, FRCS*

KEYWORDS

- Image-guided • Hybrid theater • Localization • Uniportal • Video-assisted thoracic surgery
- Hook wire • Electromagnetic navigation bronchoscopy

KEY POINTS

- Uniportal thoracoscopic surgery is a minimally invasive option for managing small pulmonary nodules and is gaining in popularity globally.
- Intraoperative nodule localization can be problematic, increasing the necessity for adjuvant localizing techniques.
- Cone-beam computed tomography has the promising ability to visualize the target lesion and its surrounding critical anatomy with an error of less than 2 mm.
- Real-time imaging helps to increase the procedural accuracy of electromagnetic navigation bronchoscopy by identifying misplacement of and guiding biopsy tools deployment.
- Centralization of the hook wire placement with simultaneous resection inside the hybrid theater may reduce wire-associated complications and provide a promising, cost-effective solution.

 Video content accompanies this article at http://www.thoracic.theclinics.com.

RATIONALE FOR LUNG NODULE MANAGEMENT IN THE HYBRID THEATER

For most of the pulmonary nodules discovered incidentally by thoracic imaging, the likelihood of them becoming malignant varies according to their size.[1] Despite the fact that small nodules tend to be benign rather than malignant, histologic diagnosis is strongly recommended for nodules that have a solid component greater than 5 mm or show enlargement on follow-up.[1] These nodules may require more invasive interventions regarding diagnosis and excision because of the low accuracy rate and false-negative biopsy samples via conventional percutaneous and bronchoscopic approaches. Furthermore, identification and excision of these small lung tumors, even by limited sublobar resections, can provide excellent prognosis.[2,3]

Disclosure: Z. Zhao and R.W.H. Lau declare no conflict of interest. C.S.H. Ng has an electromagnetic navigational bronchoscopy system SuperDimension Version 7 on loan from Medtronic.
Division of Cardiothoracic Surgery, Department of Surgery, The Chinese University of Hong Kong, Prince of Wales Hospital, Shatin, N.T., Hong Kong SAR, China
* Corresponding author.
E-mail address: calvinng@surgery.cuhk.edu.hk

Thorac Surg Clin 27 (2017) 347–355
http://dx.doi.org/10.1016/j.thorsurg.2017.06.003
1547-4127/17/© 2017 Elsevier Inc. All rights reserved.

Single-port, or uniportal, video-assisted thoracic surgery (VATS), which is gaining popularity worldwide,[4–8] may be even more problematic for localizing pulmonary lesions. The single intercostal access not only causes instrument fencing[9] but could also significantly limit surgeons from effectively palpating lesions, especially when lesions are located away from the single incision, at a distance from the pleural surface or those presenting as part-solid lesions with high ground-glass opacity (GGO).[10] Therefore, preoperative adjunctive localization techniques such as hookwire/microcoil placement or dye labeling conducted under computed tomography (CT) guidance have been widely used for identifying pulmonary lesions.

Nevertheless, these approaches inevitably increase the cost, complication, and complexity of care, all of which lead to a considerable logistic burden. The use of a hybrid operating room (OR) that can localize and manage an undetermined nodule in one suite would save time and cost, for example, by reducing hospital admissions, as well as reduce the rate of pneumothorax, marker dislodgement, and dye diffusion. Thus, a less invasive diagnostic and therapeutic option for patients could be provided.

PERFORMANCE OF INTRAOPERATIVE COMPUTED TOMOGRAPHY

When compared with conventional gantry-sized multidetector CT (MDCT), cone-beam CT (CBCT) has the advantage of multiaxis scanning, which is vital when off-plane access paths are required (eg, decubitus, semisupine).[11] The CBCT has been shown to offer equivalent accuracy to that of MDCT guidance for the transthoracic needle biopsy of lung nodules (96% vs 94%),[12] while maintaining similar effective dose, overall procedural time, and acceptable number of needle corrections.[13]

Modern mobile CBCT can provide submillimeter spatial resolution combined with soft tissue visibility even at a low radiation dose ($\sim$4.3 mGy per scan) for thoracic spine surgery.[14] However, the residual air in the collapsed lungs can make the visibility of pulmonary nodules in CBCT quite challenging. In 2013, Uneri and colleagues[15] proposed the 2-step deformable image registration for intraoperative CBCT to guide the targeting of small lesions in 12 porcine specimens under VATS. This study provided new insights into centralizing the localization, diagnosis, and treatment procedures in a hybrid OR. In detail, a robust model-driven method was used to match the pleural surface and bronchial structures between lung inflation

and deflation, achieving a coarse localization of the target wedge with an associated error of less than 3 to 5 mm. Subsequently, a finer image-driven stage that used an intensity-corrected algorithm was used to decrease the registration error to 1 to 2 mm for both the target and surrounding critical structures.

The geometric accuracy quantified by the target registration error in the anatomic targets was 1.9 mm (95% confidence interval [CI] maximum = 5.0 mm) for the initial stage, and 0.6 mm (95% CI maximum = 4.1 mm) for the subsequent stage. Moreover, with a slightly increased dose ($\sim$4.6–11.1 mGy), the scan protocol demonstrated good visibility in deflated lung tissue. Therefore, clinicians would be confident in identifying a lesion regardless of its radiological density (eg, GGO) and could evaluate potential handicaps in the hybrid OR; for instance, whether there is a bronchus sign that indicates a direct route for biopsy via bronchoscopy, or if there are any adjacent vascular structures one should be aware of during percutaneous puncture.

Preoperative CT imaging could also be incorporated into the intraoperative CBCT, which may potentially provide intraoperative segmentation anatomy for a target lesion by aligning preoperative planning with on-table data.[16]

SETTING UP A HYBRID THEATER

The integration of real-time on-table image guidance technology into clinical practice is well established in other specialties, including cardiovascular and orthopedic surgery. Anecdotal reports of the use of a portable CBCT device to detect pulmonary lesions[17] have helped to inform the use of the hybrid technique in the field of thoracic surgery, although the technique may have shortcomings in that it lacks a predetermined scanning field, which may potentially lead to an increase in intraoperative radiation exposure.[10] The idea has also been tested in pediatric surgery.[18] The first comprehensive hybrid suite and procedural flow for thoracic surgery were introduced by the Brigham and Women's Hospital group in 2013, with the Advanced Multimodal Image-Guided Operating (AMIGO) suite[19] for image-guided VATS (iVATS). The 5700-square-feet AMIGO suite has 3 separate but integrated rooms that incorporate CT, MRI, near-infrared imaging, and PET, offering great assistance in the multidisciplinary treatment of a variety of diseases.

A relatively smaller suite (approximately 760 square feet) was established in the authors' hospital.[20,21] This OR also implemented a multidisciplinary design and had proven capable of image-guided electromagnetic navigation bronchoscopy (ENB)[22] and VATS procedures, including the single-port approach.[20] The high flexibility of the floor-mounted devices allows them to be moved quickly from a distant parked position to the surgical field without interfering with the laminar airflow; thus, the OR can be highly used for multidisciplinary work. The detailed contents of the hybrid OR are described in **Box 1**.

IMAGE-GUIDED ELECTROMAGNETIC NAVIGATION BRONCHOSCOPY PROCEDURES IN THE HYBRID OPERATING ROOM

As one of the most advanced bronchoscopic techniques, ENB uses electromagnetic sensor technology in combination with virtual 3-dimensional (3D) bronchial reconstruction of CT images that can be paired with the real bronchoscopic images.[23] Once the tip of the localization guide approaches the proximity of the lesion during the navigational phase, the localization guide will then be withdrawn, leaving the extended working channel (EWC) locked onto the bronchoscope. Physicians are then able to deliver a steerable catheter for biopsy or to insert markers. The mean accuracy of the navigation system, measured by the "average fiducial target registration error" (AFTRE), defined as the distance between the marked structures on the planning CT images and the registration points recorded by bronchoscopy, was reported to range from 2.85 to 9.53 mm (mean, 6.12 mm; SD, 1.7 mm) in a pilot study (n = 30).[24] Another study with a larger

---

Box 1
Configurations of the hybrid operation room for image-guided thoracic surgery (Prince of Wales Hospital, Hong Kong)

Artis zeego multi-axis robotic imaging system (Siemens Healthcare AG, Forchheim, Germany)

Free-floating Artis OR table

Large display mounted on rails

syngo X Workplace (Siemens Healthcare AG, Forchheim, Germany)

Steris OR lamps

Dräger anesthetic workplace

Dräger Motiva supply unit

Olympus and Storz 2D and 3D endoscopic systems

Medtronic superDimension Navigation System (Covidien, Minneapolis, MN, USA)

2.5-m × 2.5-m (8.2-ft × 8.2-ft) laminar airflow field

---

number of enrolled cases (n = 92) showed that the mean AFTRE was 9 ± 6 mm (range, 1–31 mm) and that the diagnostic yield was independent of lesion size.[25] Indeed, it was suggested that an AFTRE of ≤4 mm would lead to a higher diagnostic accuracy (77.2% vs 44.4%; $P = 0.03$).[26] It should, however, be noted that these studies were based on systems and software that are a decade or more old.

The navigational error may explain the results from a recent multi-institutional study that included 581 patients, in which the diagnostic yield of the ENB technique alone was 38.5%, which was lower than previous studies that ranged from 68% to 71% when combined with radial probe endobronchial ultrasound (EBUS) or fluoroscopic guidance.[27] One argument was that continuous biopsy hits, with limited variation, were of limited added value with regard to target examination when the EWC diverged from the target, leading to a so-called all or none phenomenon. Usually, fluoroscopy or EBUS is used to indicate the position of the sensor probe in real time. However, such methods do not obviate the fundamental problem of the navigational error: one cannot be sure whether the tip of the catheter is inside the difficult-to-reach lesion. Perhaps more importantly, the movement of the EWC from the torque exerted during deployment of the biopsy tool could also contribute significantly to navigation biopsy error.

To further improve the accuracy and applicability of this technology, he authors recently reported the use of integrated CBCT (syngo dynaCT; Siemens Healthcare AG, Forchheim, Germany) and ENB in a hybrid OR, providing unparalleled real-time images to guide and confirm the successful navigation to, and biopsy of, a subcentimeter lesion located peripherally within the right middle lobe.[22] Briefly, the navigation system is switched off after the EWC has been anchored according to the guiding plan with the biopsy tool deployed, and then the Artis zeego multi-axis robotic imaging system (Siemens Healthcare AG, Forchheim, Germany) is moved to the working system without altering the position of the patient. A 6-s suspension of ventilation allows the intraoperative dynaCT to visualize the current biopsy tools and lesion. A nonmetallic device mounted on the table is used to hold the bronchoscope still during scanning (**Fig. 1**). Normally, 2 intraoperative scans are required: one to identify any minor misdirection and the second to confirm the biopsy after any necessary adjustment has taken place. To further decrease the exposure to radiation, 2 fluoroscopic shots taken from different angles by the dynaCT can orientate the catheter after 2-dimensional

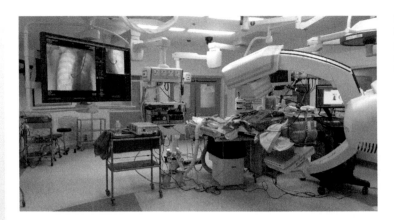

Fig. 1. Hybrid theater with CBCT image-guided electromagnetic navigation bronchoscopy (iENB) at Prince of Wales Hospital, The Chinese University of Hong Kong.

(2D)/3D fusion with the preoperative CT data; thus, the radiation dose is comparable to a preoperative percutaneous biopsy. The image from the dynaCT in the hybrid OR reveals its superior accuracy over fluoroscopy or EBUS in determining the direction of the catheter tip, because it provides undisputable evidence of the tip and tool reaching their target (**Fig. 2**; Video 1). Hence, the navigational error can be decreased, particularly when dealing with GGO lesions of less than 10 mm that are poorly visualized on standard fluoroscopy and EBUS. Thus far, the authors have applied this technique to 12 patients with lesion size ranging from 8 mm to 39 mm (median, 22 mm), and 5 of them were pure GGO. No complication was met, and 83.3% diagnostic yield was achieved in their series.[28]

In addition, this ultraprecise diagnostic procedure through ENB could be of great importance when dealing with multifocal pulmonary lesions. For example, through rapid on-site evaluation or

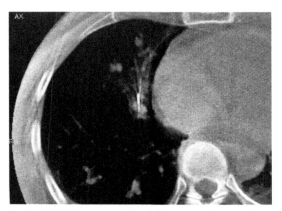

Fig. 2. CBCT image provide definitive evidence of successful navigation and intervention by the ENB, in this case of a subcentimeter right middle lobe lesion.

frozen section,[29] the surgeon may choose a sublobar resection or even from a range of endoscopic therapies that are in development (eg, ablation, cryotherapy) for a marginally malignant lesion in a particular segment while performing an anatomic lobectomy for an invasive cancer in an adjacent lobe in order to preserve pulmonary function. Such complex and tailored management may have an increasingly important role in treatment of early detected cancer and for an aging population.[30]

Recently, Marino and colleagues[31] reported the largest series to date on ENB-guided transbronchial injection of dye followed by VATS sublobar resection in a conventional OR. Of the 72 pulmonary nodules that ranged in size from 4 to 17 mm (median, 8 mm), 70 were successfully identified without complication. In their technique, one dose of methylene blue (<0.5 mL) was injected into the nodule and another shot was given to mark the pleura if the nodule was located more than 5 mm from the pleural surface. One case experienced dye extravasation but was palpated intraoperatively. Undoubtedly, the hybrid technique would allow for more precise placement of marking dye in close proximity to lesions for resection margin guidance under single-port VATS, representing a future direction for this technology (**Figs. 3** and **4**).[32]

IMAGE-GUIDED PERCUTANEOUS LOCALIZATION IN THE HYBRID OPERATING ROOM

The preoperative implantation of a radiopaque metallic material such as a hook wire or microcoil under CT guidance has been adopted by many thoracic surgeons and has provided a high level of evidence for the efficacy of intraoperative localization, although there is a slightly lower

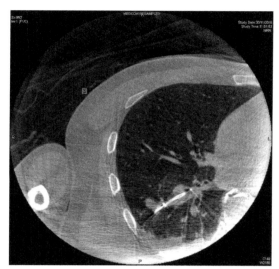

Fig. 3. Hybrid theater CBCT-guided iENB methylene blue dye marking of right lower lobe lesion showing the injection needle deployed adjacent to the target.

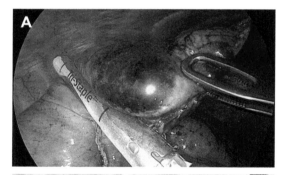

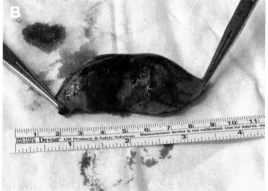

Fig. 4. (A) One-stop immediate uniportal VATS resection of the iENB marked lesion in the hybrid theater, (B) resected lung with dye marking at the pleural surface and adjacent to subcentimeter nodule.

successful operative field targeting rate due to dislodgement or migration compared with lipiodol or microcoil localization.[33,34] The drawback of a lack of tactile sense during single-port VATS can be compensated for by visualizing these metallic materials with part of the filament left outside the pleural surface or detected through intraoperative fluoroscopy. Also, gentle extrathoracic manipulation of the outer filament of the wire tail may allow for traction of the lung nodule in directions that would facilitate VATS resection.[35]

Classically, these techniques require localization to be performed in the radiology suite followed by surgery in the conventional OR. During the time incurred in transporting patients to the OR, patients might experience discomfort and suffer from various complications such as pneumothorax or dislodgement of the localizing material.[10] Approximately 24% of patients who undergo hook-wire insertion are likely to experience pneumothorax, and 2% to 4% of them may require chest tube drainage before surgery. Wire dislodgement from the mounting pleura remains the major factor (2%–10%) in the failure of localization, which is a higher rate than for microcoil implantation (2.7%).[33] However, the pneumothorax rate associated with the microcoil cannot be ignored, which has been reported to be as high as 13%, although a chest tube was rarely needed in these cases.[36]

As discussed above, the iVATS program proposed by the Brigham and Women's Hospital group attempted to simultaneously centralize the implantation procedure with subsequent surgery in the AMIGO theater and showed this technique to be advantageous compared with conducting these procedures separately. In their phase 1-2 study, 23 pulmonary lesions of size 1.30 ± 0.38 cm received conventional thoracoscopic surgery after the placement of 2 T-shaped fiducials (Kimberly-Clark, Roswell, GA, USA) under intraoperative C-arm CT.[37] A 5-s end-inspiratory-hold 200° rotation with a 0.36 mGy per projection scanning protocol for the predetermined field was able to identify the nodule by CBCT. Two T-bar fiducials were implanted afterward for localization under fluoroscopic guidance according to the trajectory provided by the syngo iGuide needle guidance software (Siemens Healthcare AG, Forchheim, Germany). Notably, the T-bars were successfully implanted in 20 (87.0%) cases, with a median procedure duration of 39 minutes. The average and total procedure radiation doses were low (median: 1501 mGy × m²; range, 665–16,326 mGy × m²). Interestingly, no implantation-associated complication was found, compared with the traditional 2-suite workflow.

Furthermore, the iVATS protocol may provide a minimally invasive service through single-port VATS, since the authors' group reported the world's first image-guided single-port VATS (iSP-VATS) major lung resection for a GGO nodule that underwent dynaCT-guided hook-wire placement in the hybrid OR.[20] Two fluoroscopic shots by the dynaCT are administered to ensure that the lesion is in the isocenter of the CBCT, and optimal tube parameters will be automatically created to provide a 3D real-time image of the thorax. On the syngo X Workplace, the interventional radiologist deploys the hook wire to the chest, and the control scans further verify the position of the needle (**Fig. 5**). Optionally, the Artis zeego can be equipped with a laser cross-indicator to aid the puncturing process under the guidance of the iGuide software mentioned above. Approximately 30 minutes is needed to localize and place a hook wire; the radiation exposure level for this procedure is comparable to the conventional percutaneous technique in the radiology suite. Pulmonary deflation after the introduction of one-lung ventilation may theoretically cause wire dislodgement, but this could also be solved immediately by relocalizing the lesion in the hybrid unit, because the CBCT can visualize the pulmonary structure in a collapsed lung.[15] The authors' hook-wire iSPVATS technique would work perfectly for peripheral lesions of even subcentimeter size and may reduce the risk of complications associated with marker implantation.

Thus far, the authors have attempted 19 consecutive cases under minimally invasive sublobar resection of small pulmonary nodules with real-time image-guided hook-wire localization in the hybrid OR between February 2014 and October 2015. The mean nodule size was 7.7 ± 3.4 mm (range: 2–15 mm), and all of them were accurately localized by hook wire and successfully resected. VATS resections were immediately performed in the hybrid OR after hook-wire insertion. Five (26.3%) patients developed pneumothorax after hook-wire insertion, but none required intervention. The mean operating time was 128.5 ± 60.6 minutes, and the average blood loss was 25.5 ± 15.0 mL. The mean chest drainage duration was 2.6 ± 0.9 days, and the postoperative length of hospital stay was 3.6 ± 1.7 days. No postoperative complications or mortality occurred. Regarding the histology, 14 (73.7%) malignant and 5 benign lesions were identified, all with adequate resection margins. This preliminary cohort showed that real-time image-guided hook-wire localization in the hybrid OR setting is a safe and effective technique for VATS resection for tiny lung nodules.[38]

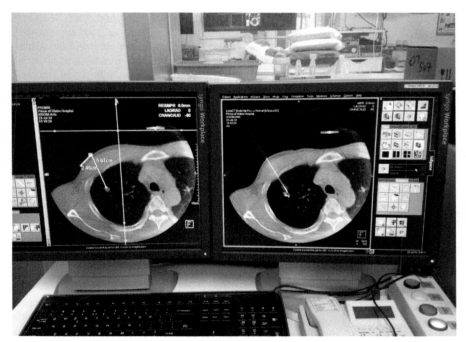

Fig. 5. CT scan viewed in the hybrid theater control room of a deep right upper lobe lesion with measurements to guide percutaneous hook-wire insertion (*left*), and a follow-up scan taken 23 minutes later after successful localization with percutaneous hook wire (*right*).

Table 1
Comparison of recent reports of image-guided localization with immediate resection under video-assisted thoracic surgery in the hybrid theater

	n	Size, mm (Median)	Localization Method	Successful Rate, %	Procedure-Associated Complication (n, %)	Localization Time	CBCT Scan Times
Gill et al[37]	23	6–18 (13)	T-fiducials implantation	87	0	39 (23–62) min	1–2
Yang et al[11]	25	5–20 (10)	Dye injection	92	Liver puncture (1, 4%) Pneumothorax (1, 4%)	46 (27–69) min	3
Yu et al[38,a]	19	2–15 (7.7)	Hook wire	100	Pneumothorax (5, 26.3%)	NA	2

Abbreviation: NA, not applicable.
[a] Part of the cases underwent uniportal VATS.

Image-guided percutaneous dye localization in the hybrid OR was also reported to be successfully performed in 23 of the 25 patients (92%) by the Taiwanese group.[11] An additional (third) dynaCT scan was acquired under the end-inspiratory hold phase to confirm immersion of the injected dye around the target, which is slightly different from the authors' protocol (**Table 1**). However, it is noteworthy that technical limitations remain in these percutaneous approaches to marking because nodules that are located near the apex, mediastinum, and diaphragm can be difficult to access. One patient with a right middle lobe lesion experienced a puncture through the diaphragm into the liver parenchyma in a previous report.[11]

FURTHER CONSIDERATIONS FOR IMPROVING THORACIC SERVICE IN HYBRID SUITE

Currently, most hybrid ORs are usually equipped with floatable angiography tables, which were originally designed for cardiovascular interventions and are not designed to be bridged. In the authors' experience, the insertion of soft support below midchest would help expand the intercostal space for most uniportal procedures when bridging is needed. It is also recommended that during the docking procedure, lines and equipment at the cranial side should be arranged properly to make sure that the CBCT could rotate freely around the patient. Furthermore, the time-schedule designing and corporation among multidisciplinary specialties is vital when starting up this program.

SUMMARY

Precise localization is of paramount importance in the management of small pulmonary lesions,

especially in the era of single port VATS. Centralization of the diagnostic and localizing procedures within a specially designed hybrid theater could enhance diagnostic accuracy as well as decrease the complications associated with percutaneous puncture. By using ENB under CBCT-guided real-time adjustment, the chance of biopsy error is reduced, consequently avoiding missing significant abnormality and unnecessary excisions particularly when dealing with multiple lesions. Dye labeling via ENB or percutaneous approach, which has recently been shown to be a powerful method for localizing small pulmonary lesions for sublobar resection, can also benefit from the hybrid OR strategy to increase marking precision and may improve resection margin accuracy. The iSPVATS concept, using a hook wire/microcoil, allows for a safer percutaneous procedure in the OR environment and minimizes the chance of dislodgement and localization failure. Moreover, the CBCT could provide salvage localization in the rare case of marker dislodgement, because it is capable of visualizing pulmonary lesions within deflated lung.

The tailored concept of minimally invasive thoracic surgery is evolving from simply reducing the number of surgical incisions, as has been seen with the development of uniportal VATS, to becoming a more sophisticated art of minimizing surgical insult to the patient by, for example, lung-preserving surgical resections through improved localization procedures, or fast-tracking using techniques such as nonintubated anesthesia.[30,39] It is anticipated that the hybrid OR will play an increasingly important role in this exciting progress as it establishes a cost-effective, one-stop procedural flow for image-guided thoracic surgery. Advanced hybrid ORs, like the AMIGO suite, which incorporate other modalities of imaging may have implications in providing additional information and details for safer and more efficient surgery of the future.

SUPPLEMENTARY DATA

Supplementary data related to this article can be found online at http://dx.doi.org/10.1016/j.thorsurg.2017.06.003.

REFERENCES

1. Naidich DP, Bankier AA, MacMahon H, et al. Recommendations for the management of subsolid pulmonary nodules detected at CT: a statement from the Fleischner Society. Radiology 2013;266(1):304–17.
2. Dai C, Shen J, Ren Y, et al. Choice of surgical procedure for patients with non-small-cell lung cancer </= 1 cm or > 1 to 2 cm among lobectomy, segmentectomy, and wedge resection: a population-based study. J Clin Oncol 2016;34(26):3175–82.
3. Zhao ZR, Situ DR, Lau RWH, et al. Comparison of segmentectomy and lobectomy in stage IA adenocarcinomas >1 and ≤2 cm: a brief report. J Thorac Oncol 2017;12(5):890–6.
4. Ng CS, Lau KK, Gonzalez-Rivas D, et al. Evolution in surgical approach and techniques for lung cancer. Thorax 2013;68(7):681.
5. Ng CS, Rocco G, Wong RH, et al. Uniportal and single-incision video-assisted thoracic surgery: the state of the art. Interact Cardiovasc Thorac Surg 2014;19(4):661–6.
6. Ng CS, Kim HK, Wong RH, et al. Single-port video-assisted thoracoscopic major lung resections: experience with 150 consecutive cases. Thorac Cardiovasc Surg 2016;64(4):348–53.
7. Zhao ZR, Li Z, Situ DR, et al. Recent clinical innovations in thoracic surgery in Hong Kong. J Thorac Dis 2016;8(Suppl 8):S618–26.
8. Gonzalez-Rivas D, Yang Y, Ng C. Advances in uniportal video-assisted thoracoscopic surgery: pushing the envelope. Thorac Surg Clin 2016;26(2):187–201.
9. Ng CS, Wong RH, Lau RW, et al. Minimizing chest wall trauma in single-port video-assisted thoracic surgery. J Thorac Cardiovasc Surg 2014;147(3):1095–6.
10. Zhao ZR, Lau RW, Ng CS. Hybrid theatre and alternative localization techniques in conventional and single-port video-assisted thoracoscopic surgery. J Thorac Dis 2016;8(Suppl 3):S319–27.
11. Yang SM, Ko WC, Lin MW, et al. Image-guided thoracoscopic surgery with dye localization in a hybrid operating room. J Thorac Dis 2016;8(Suppl 9):S681–9.
12. Rotolo N, Floridi C, Imperatori A, et al. Comparison of cone-beam CT-guided and CT fluoroscopy-guided transthoracic needle biopsy of lung nodules. Eur Radiol 2016;26(2):381–9.
13. Kostrzewa M, Rathmann N, Kara K, et al. Accuracy of percutaneous soft-tissue interventions using a multi-axis, C-arm CT system and 3D laser guidance. Eur J Radiol 2015;84(10):1970–5.
14. Schafer S, Nithiananthan S, Mirota DJ, et al. Mobile C-arm cone-beam CT for guidance of spine surgery: image quality, radiation dose, and integration with interventional guidance. Med Phys 2011;38(8):4563–74.
15. Uneri A, Nithiananthan S, Schafer S, et al. Deformable registration of the inflated and deflated lung in cone-beam CT-guided thoracic surgery: initial investigation of a combined model- and image-driven approach. Med Phys 2013;40(1):017501.
16. Nithiananthan S, Schafer S, Uneri A, et al. Demons deformable registration of CT and cone-beam CT using an iterative intensity matching approach. Med Phys 2011;38(4):1785–98.
17. Ohtaka K, Takahashi Y, Kaga K, et al. Video-assisted thoracoscopic surgery using mobile computed tomography: new method for locating of small lung nodules. J Cardiothorac Surg 2014;9:110.
18. Narayanam S, Gerstle T, Amaral J, et al. Lung tattooing combined with immediate video-assisted thoracoscopic resection (IVATR) as a single procedure in a hybrid room: our institutional experience in a pediatric population. Pediatr Radiol 2013;43(9):1144–51.
19. Advanced Multimodality Image Guided Operating (AMIGO). 2016. Available at: http://www.brighamandwomens.org/research/amigo/default.aspx. Accessed November 29, 2016.
20. Ng CS, Man Chu C, Kwok MW, et al. Hybrid DynaCT scan-guided localization single-port lobectomy. [corrected]. Chest 2015;147(3):e76–8.
21. Zhao ZR, Lau RWH, Yu PSY, et al. Image-guided localization of small lung nodules in video-assisted thoracic surgery. J Thorac Dis 2016;8(Suppl 9):S731–7.
22. Ng CS, Yu SC, Lau RW, et al. Hybrid DynaCT-guided electromagnetic navigational bronchoscopic biopsy†. Eur J Cardiothorac Surg 2016;49(Suppl 1):i87–8.
23. Schwarz Y, Mehta AC, Ernst A, et al. Electromagnetic navigation during flexible bronchoscopy. Respiration 2003;70(5):516–22.
24. Becker HD, Herth F, Ernst A, et al. Bronchoscopic biopsy of peripheral lung lesions under electromagnetic guidance: a pilot study. J Bronchol 2005;12(1):9–13.
25. Eberhardt R, Anantham D, Herth F, et al. Electromagnetic navigation diagnostic bronchoscopy in peripheral lung lesions. Chest 2007;131(6):1800–5.

26. Makris D, Scherpereel A, Leroy S, et al. Electromagnetic navigation diagnostic bronchoscopy for small peripheral lung lesions. Eur Respir J 2007;29(6): 1187–92.

27. Ost DE, Ernst A, Lei X, et al. Diagnostic yield and complications of bronchoscopy for peripheral lung lesions. results of the AQuIRE registry. Am J Respir Crit Care Med 2016;193(1):68–77.

28. Lau WH, Chow CYS, Ho YKJ, et al. Hybrid operating room dynaCT real-time image guided electromagnetic navigation bronchoscopic biospy (iENB) - the initial experience. Respirology 2016;21(Suppl. 3):74.

29. Iding JS, Krimsky W, Browning R. Tissue requirements in lung cancer diagnosis for tumor heterogeneity, mutational analysis and targeted therapies: initial experience with intra-operative Frozen Section Evaluation (FROSE) in bronchoscopic biopsies. J Thorac Dis 2016;8(Suppl 6):S488–93.

30. Ng CSH, Zhao ZR, Lau RWH. Tailored therapy for stage I non–small-cell lung cancer. J Clin Oncol 2017;35(3):268–70.

31. Marino KA, Sullivan JL, Weksler B. Electromagnetic navigation bronchoscopy for identifying lung nodules for thoracoscopic resection. Ann Thorac Surg 2016;102(2):454–7.

32. Rocco R, Rocco G. Future study direction on single port (uniportal) VATS. J Thorac Dis 2016;8(Suppl 3): S328–32.

33. Kidane B, Yasufuku K. Advances in image-guided thoracic surgery. Thorac Surg Clin 2016;26(2): 129–38.

34. Park CH, Han K, Hur J, et al. Comparative effectiveness and safety of pre-operative lung localization for pulmonary nodules: a systematic review and meta-analysis. Chest 2016. http://dx.doi.org/10.1016/j.chest.2016.09.017. Accessed December 17, 2016.

35. Ng CS, Hui JW, Wong RH. Minimizing single-port access in video-assisted wedge resection, with a hookwire. Asian Cardiovasc Thorac Ann 2013; 21(1):114–5.

36. Finley RJ, Mayo JR, Grant K, et al. Preoperative computed tomography-guided microcoil localization of small peripheral pulmonary nodules: a prospective randomized controlled trial. J Thorac Cardiovasc Surg 2015;149(1):26–31.

37. Gill RR, Zheng Y, Barlow JS, et al. Image-guided video assisted thoracoscopic surgery (iVATS) - phase I-II clinical trial. J Surg Oncol 2015;112(1): 18–25.

38. Yu PS, Lau RW, Capili GF, et al. Minimally-invasive sublobar resection of tiny pulmonary nodules with real-time image guidance in the hybrid theatre. Innovations 2016;11:S98–9.

39. Zhao ZR, Lau RWH, Ng CSH. Non-intubated video-assisted thoracic surgery: the final frontier? Eur J Cardiothorac Surg 2016;50(5):925–6.

Important Technical Details During Uniportal Video-Assisted Thoracoscopic Major Resections

CrossMark

Diego Gonzalez-Rivas, MD, FECTS[a,b,c,*],
Alan D.L. Sihoe, MBBChir, MA(Cantab), FRCSEd(CTh), FCSHK, FHKAM, FCCP[d,e,f,g]

KEYWORDS

- VATS • Single port VATS • Uniportal VATS • Lobectomy • Operative setup • Instrumentation

KEY POINTS

- Since it was first performed in 2010, lobectomy via a single port—uniportal video-assisted thoracoscopic surgery (VATS)—has become increasingly popular among surgeons.
- The uniportal approach requires a different skill set compared to conventional VATS. The parallel instrumentation achieved through this access mimics the maneuvers performed during open surgery.
- Surgeons experienced with a 2-port technique or with anterior thoracotomy approach will probably adopt the uniportal concept faster.

 Video content accompanies this article at http://www.thoracic.theclinics.com.

INTRODUCTION

Since the first uniportal video-assisted thoracoscopic surgery (VATS) major pulmonary resection was performed in 2010,[1] the technique has been spreading worldwide.[2–4] As with other minimally invasive approaches, the uniportal VATS technique for all patients with resectable lung cancer follows the oncological principles of open surgery by anatomic dissection of individual vascular and bronchial structures, and by complete radical lymphadenectomy.[5]

The uniportal approach allows a direct visualization of the target tissue and of the pulmonary hilum from the front side. The parallel instrumentation achieved through this access mimics the maneuvers performed during open surgery, and this makes the movements of the surgeon more comfortable.[6–8] Therefore, surgeons experienced with the 2-port technique or with the anterior thoracotomy approach will probably adopt the uniportal concept more readily than those surgeons more used to the 3-port technique.

Because only 1 intercostal space is involved without rib spreading or muscle disruption, and because the incision is usually placed more anteriorly than with conventional VATS, some authors reported less postoperative pain, faster

[a] Uniportal VATS Training Program, Shanghai Pulmonary Hospital, Shanghai, China; [b] Departments of Thoracic Surgery and Lung Transplantation, Coruña University Hospital, Coruña, Spain; [c] Minimally Invasive Thoracic Surgery Unit (UCTMI), Coruña, Spain; [d] Department of Surgery, The University of Hong Kong, Hong Kong; [e] The University of Hong Kong Shenzhen Hospital, Shenzhen, China; [f] Department of Thoracic Surgery, Tongji University, Shanghai Pulmonary Hospital, Shanghai, China; [g] Cardiothoracic Surgery Unit, Queen Mary Hospital, Hong Kong
* Corresponding author. Department of Thoracic Surgery, Coruña University Hospital, Xubias 84, Coruña 15006, Spain.
E-mail address: diego.gonzalez.rivas@sergas.es

Thorac Surg Clin 27 (2017) 357–372
http://dx.doi.org/10.1016/j.thorsurg.2017.06.004
1547-4127/17/© 2017 Elsevier Inc. All rights reserved.

postoperative recovery, reduced duration of hospital stay, and potentially earlier administration of adjuvant therapy when necessary.[9,10]

However, there are several important technical details that must be learned to achieve successful outcomes. In this article, we analyze some common difficulties that thoracic surgeons could find in their common practice of this technique. We provide practical tips and tricks, and summarize the most important technical details to accomplish optimal exposure for an oncologic procedure.

GENERAL ASPECTS AND BASIC SURGICAL PRINCIPLES
Evolution in Instrumentation and Camera Placement

In recent years, the uniportal technique has evolved considerably, not only in the growing range of complex cases performed, but also in the fine details of the instrumentation. Initially, when we described the technique in 2010, the camera was not always in the same position within the uniport and multiple instruments often had to be used via the uniport at the same time because dedicated uniportal instruments were not then available.[1] The result was constant interference and fencing with the camera. Also, the incision was of a larger size (4–5 cm) to accommodate the multiple instruments.

Thanks to gained experience, the introduction of bespoke instruments and improvement in the image systems, we have refined the technique to produce a concept called "advanced instrumentation." It consists of simplifying the instrumentation using the fewest number of instruments: most of the surgery is now performed using a long, curved suction device in the left hand, and an energy device in the right hand. The shape of the long, curved suction device is ideally suited for use via

a small uniport, allowing compression of structures, blunt dissection, retraction of tissues, and even support and movement of the lymph node package during lymphadenectomy. A dedicated endoscopic surgery energy device (using ultrasonic and/or diathermy energy) is fantastic, and can be used to dissect vessels, retract tissues, coagulate and cut structures, and even grasp organs in some occasions. This evolution in the instrumentation has allowed the size of the incision to be reduced considerably (2–3 cm at present) without interfering with the operating time or results (**Fig. 1**).

Experience also now confirms that one of the basic principles of uniportal VATS is to keep the camera always located at the top of the incision, and to introduce the instruments and staplers below the camera via the lower part of the wound.[11] Because human eyes are normally above the level of the hands, this arrangement allows for a more natural and ergonomic surgery: the camera provides a "top-down" view of the operative field, and the instruments are visualized coming into the field from the lower sides of the monitor view.

How to Localize the Correct Intercostal Space: Tips About the Incision

As a routine, the best location is usually in the fifth intercostal space, between the mid and anterior axillary lines.[11] For upper lobectomies—especially on the left—an incision that is too high (fourth intercostal space) gives a difficult angle for the insertion of the stapler for superior pulmonary vein division. The slightly anterior position of the incision provides a more anatomic instrumentation for the surgeon standing in front of the patient, and reduces the possibility of postoperative pain because of the naturally wider intercostal space anteriorly. On the right side, the fifth intercostal space

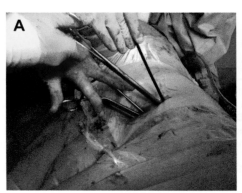
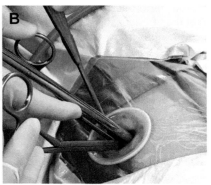

Fig. 1. External view of surgical technique during (*A*) the early period (2010), and (*B*) after 7 years of experience using advanced instrumentation (2017).

remains the best location for right middle and lower lobectomies, but with experience the fourth intercostal space is normally used for right upper lobectomies. On the left side, the fifth intercostal space should always be used for all resections, and the incision should be slightly more lateral to avoid interference of the view and instrumentation by the beating heart.

It should be noted, however, that even among experienced uniportal VATS surgeons, there can be slight variations in the siting of the incision. Some would prefer a slightly more posterior location near the midaxillary line, allowing a posterior-to-anterior hilar dissection.[12] Nevertheless, a more anterior incision is preferable for most patients, and is certainly the recommended option for beginners.

The size of the incision depends on the experience of the surgeon, but during the learning curve should not be too large (not more than 6 cm, because the camera and the instruments lose points of support) or too small (not smaller than 3 cm, because interference and fencing between instruments can occur). The incision itself is typically 3 to 4 cm long, although longer incisions can be used for large tumors, for complex procedures, and for a patient who is obese or has a thick chest wall. A longer incision has not been shown to cause any obvious disadvantage to the patient.[5,13]

The incision is made according to muscle-sparing technique principles: the 2 bellies of the serratus muscle are opened without cutting the fibers and then the intercostal muscle is cut along the upper edge of the lower rib, preserving its fibers and avoiding neural bundle injury.

When using a wound protector, it is advisable to add a lubricant oil or gel to the outside ring, because this facilitates the insertion of the instruments and reduces friction during instrumentation. In case of chest wall adhesions, it is recommended to release the most anterior or posterior adhesions before inserting the wound protector because its inside ring can restrict instruments from reaching those adhesions. As an alternative to a wound protector, the subcutaneous tissue and skin can be held open with stay sutures to the drapes. Use of a wound protector or these stay sutures is important to keep the uniport open; otherwise, use of suction inside the chest would inflate the lungs and block surgery. This is especially true in obese patients.

At the end of the operation, a single chest tube is placed via the uniport, usually at the upper part of the incision (20-F or 24-F). The drainage should be placed inside the chest cavity in a curved shape, along the costovertebral sinus, with its tip toward the apex. This position allows for both good reexpansion of the lung and effective drainage of postoperative pleural effusion. The wound is then closed in layers around the chest tube in the same manner as for the utility incision in conventional VATS. Meticulous closure, avoiding gaps between the layers, is important to prevent subcutaneous emphysema, which can develop as intrathoracic air sometimes escapes out along the chest tube tract.[5,11]

Position of the Assistant

Coordination with the assistant is very important to maintain proper instrumentation and avoid interference between the camera and instruments. When we initially described the technique, the assistant was always positioned on the same side as the surgeon, that is, anterior to the lateral decubitus patient.[11] However, increasing experience has shown that, for the upper lobes, positioning the assistant on the opposite side to the surgeon (behind the patient) has advantages for both. In this way, the surgeon has more space to work and the assistant can more easily keep the camera at the top of the uniport (**Fig. 2**A). For lower lobectomies and especially for subcarinal lymphadenectomy, management of the camera from the opposite side is very difficult, so having the assistant located on the same side as the surgeon is still recommended to allow better following of the surgeon's movements. When the first operator works on the lower part of the thorax, the assistant stands on the cranial side of patient[6] (**Fig. 2**B).

The assistant should hold the camera with the right hand or the left according to his or her position with respect to the surgeon to give the surgeon more space for action. The assistant's other hand should be prepared to help the surgeon in holding or moving the instruments when necessary.

If 2 monitors are used, each one will be placed on both sides of the patient. If only one is used, it should be at the patient's head (see **Fig. 2**). The screen should be placed at a suitable height, to avoid poor neck postures and maintain ergonomics throughout the surgery. Ideally, the middle point of the screen should be at the level of the surgeon's eyes.

Because it is important to keep the camera always located at the top of the wound, various tricks or strategies can be used to accomplish this—such as using a suture, vessel loop, or a tape that holds the camera and keeps it fixed (**Fig. 3**). In this way, we reduce the possibility of fatigue of the assistant and we assure greater stability in the vision during the surgery.

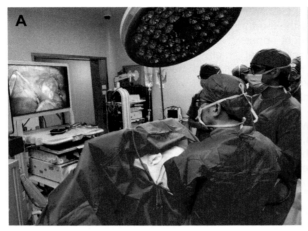
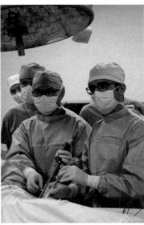

Fig. 2. Position of the assistant during (*A*) right upper lobectomy and (*B*) right lower lobectomy.

The "Rule of the Flexed Arms" for Staplers

One of the greatest difficulties during the learning curve is to know what angulation is required for the staplers, especially in the upper lobectomies. Finding out which is the best angle for the stapler insertion is time consuming and can be a cause of insecurity for beginners. There is a very simple trick called "the rule of the flexed arms" that helps us to know which angulation we should use in each lobectomy.

During lobectomy, we can dissect the lobe from the hilum first or from the fissure first. We must consider every lobe as circle with 1 curved side on the right and an opposite curved side on the left. To understand this trick is simple: we extend our arms flexed and joint in front of the screen, like we are wrapping the lobe according to the lobectomy we are performing. The stapler will always follow the direction of the arm; for example, on the right side, the upper lobe would be to the right part of the screen (our right arm) and the

lower lobe would be on the left side (our left arm). On the left side, the upper lobe will be on the left part of the screen (our left arm) and the lower will be on the right side of the screen (our right arm) (Video 1). The angles of the staplers follow the direction of the arms, according the lobe we are operating on (**Fig. 4**).

For example, for a right upper lobe, if we approach the lobe for vein and artery dissection in a hilum-first approach, we must retract the lobe in a caudal direction, and then the angle of the stapler will follow the direction of the curved right arm. If we approach the right upper lobe with a fissure-first approach, the lobe is retracted in a cranial direction, and the angle for the stapler follows the curve of our left arm, with the anvil oriented to the apex. On the left side, for a left upper lobectomy, the stapler is curved downward (following the left arm) to reach the vessels from a hilum-first approach (see **Fig. 4**A; Video 1), and if we approach the fissure the stapler is curved

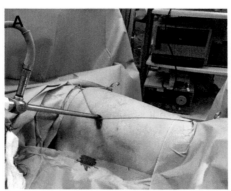
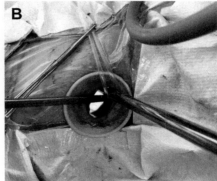

Fig. 3. Tricks to keep the camera located always in the upper part of the incision using a vessel loop (*A*) or a plastic traction (*B*).

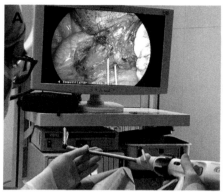
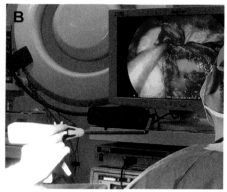

Fig. 4. The "rule of the flexed arms" for staplers during a left upper lobectomy. (*A*) When we approach the upper lobe from the hilum, the lobe must be retracted caudally and the curve of the stapler must be with the anvil oriented to the lower lobe. (*B*) When we approach the left upper lobe from the fissure, the lobe must be retracted cranially and the stapler inserted with the anvil oriented to the apex.

upward, oriented to the apex (see **Fig. 4**B). For right and left lower lobes, exactly the same concept is applied.

This trick helps to not waste time thinking about what angle is needed for every lobe. It is recommended that, before starting the surgery, the nurse assistant is informed to prepare all staplers with the angulation according this rule.

The staplers should always be inserted from the bottom of the wound, allowing the skin and the subcutaneous tissue to support and stabilize the endostapler.

The Suction Device Trick

When performing advanced instrumentation, the long, curved suction device becomes a crucial instrument with multiple functions such as to aspirate, hold, expose, compress, release adhesions, and so on. One of the basic principles of the uniportal technique is that the instruments must be curved to avoid interference with the visual field. In general, straight instruments are not suitable

for uniportal VATS. The use of a disposable plastic suction device is not recommended if an ultrasonic energy device is also used during the same operation. This caveat is because the tip can be melted, generating a sharp edge that can injure the vessels during dissection, especially if it goes unnoticed.

There is a very useful trick called "the suction device trick" when stapling the upper pulmonary vein and upper lobe bronchus.[6] Once we have performed the dissection of the vein or bronchus, we keep the dissector open wide behind the vessel and pass the long, curved suction device through that space. Then we must remove the dissector and retract the vein or bronchus upward with the suction device, creating a path through which the stapler is introduced while protecting the artery that is just behind it (see Video 1; **Fig. 5**). When stapling the right upper lobe bronchus, this trick protects possible damage of A2, and when stapling the left upper lobe bronchus with a fissureless technique, this trick protects the lingular artery (**Fig. 6**; see Video 2). This maneuver is not

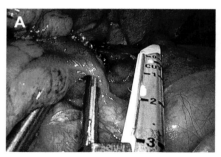
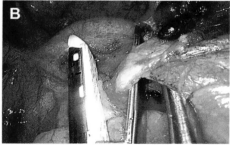

Fig. 5. The trick of the suction device to help the division of right upper pulmonary vein (*A*) and left upper pulmonary vein (*B*).

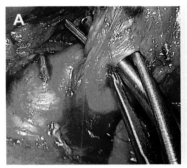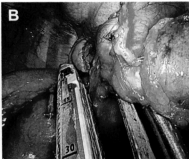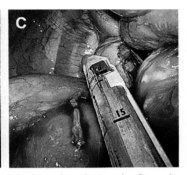

Fig. 6. The trick of the suction device to help the division of the left upper lobe bronchus during the fissureles technique. (*A*) Dissection of bronchus. (*B*) Insertion of stapler under the guidance of the suction device. (*C*) Visualization of the tip of the anvil of stapler for a safe bronchial division.

recommended for stapling of an artery because the traction of an artery could produce a hematoma or even an avulsion.

OPERATIVE TECHNIQUE: BASIC CONCEPTS

The most important thing in uniportal VATS is exposure, so the tips and tricks for this are more important than for other VATS approaches. Because there is only 1 hole, the small details and tricks represent big steps in improving exposure. It is important to use a 30° high-definition video thoracoscope and long, curved instruments designed for uniportal VATS, with proximal and distal articulation to prevent fencing and allow their simultaneous use. To achieve good instrumentation with no interference, the ideal is to keep a minimum distance of 2 cm between the camera and the instruments. The shorter this distance, the more limited the freedom of movement is and the more interference increases.

We recommend to retract only on the lobe to be resected and not on the remaining lung. It is also possible to use the sucker or a sponge-stick to help retract the lung away; these devices are less traumatic, although they provide less directional control of the retraction.

The surgical technique is completely different for upper and lower lobes. The instrumentation for lower lobes is similar to conventional VATS, where the staplers are introduced regularly through the utility incision. For upper lobes, we need to perform a different exposure and follow different strategies when compared with conventional VATS (where staplers are often introduced from a posterior port). We have 2 options to deal with the hilum according with the distance located between the upper lobe vein and artery. When the distance between both structures is long enough (artery not hidden by the vein), we can follow the first option, which is to dissect and divide the

vein first, and then the artery. However, when the distance is too short, or the angle for stapler insertion is not optimal for the vein, the recommended strategy is to dissect and divide the artery first and then the vein. On the right side, the division of the vein first usually is more difficult compared to the left side, because the incision used may be at the fourth intercostal space and the vein often hides the main artery. On the left side, usually there is more distance between the upper lobe vein and main artery, and the location of the incision also allows a more favorable angle for staplers to approach and divide the upper vein.

To divide an incomplete fissure, the artery can be exposed by dissecting upward from the hilum, first through the space between upper and lower veins, and then between upper and lower bronchus. The creation of a safe plane in a tunnel view (we can use a dissector or an energy device), allows the anvil of the stapler to be placed over the artery, dividing the anterior portion of the fissure (**Fig. 7**).

The vein is one of the critical points during uniportal VATS upper lobectomies. A stapler with a roticulating head and curved tip makes the stapling much easier, especially for the upper vein. The thinner anvil jaw of the stapler is inserted along the caudal side of upper lobe vein. If the stapler is continued to be inserted straight in, the anvil will impact on the structures behind (notably the pulmonary artery, especially if it has not been previously divided) and stapling cannot be accomplished. Therefore, once the anvil is engaged at the caudal side of the vein, the lung is retracted forward and in a cranial direction. This movement opens up space behind the vein, between it and the artery behind it. At the same time, the stapler is also gently rotated in a cranial direction so that the reticulated head is not pointing straight into the hilum, but instead is pointing in a more cranial direction. We call this maneuver the rotation trick

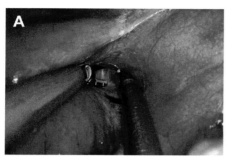
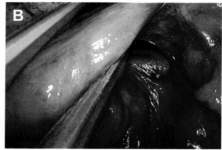

Fig. 7. Surgical image during a right lower lobectomy showing the tunnel view to expose the pulmonary artery (*A*) and the stapler inserted above the surface of basal trunk of pulmonary artery (*B*).

(**Fig. 8**). Combining this with the suction device trick facilitates the insertion of the staplers during upper vein division (see **Fig. 5** and Video 3).

If a vessel to be divided is small (up to 1 cm) and there is no good angle for a stapler, polymer vascular clips may be used. We find that a 45° clip applier designed for uniportal VATs is enormously useful. This angulation allows the surgeon to see the lock on the closing part of the clip, which makes clip deployment much safer. It is important to check that the clip engages the entire circumference of the vessel before closing to avoid any vascular damage (**Fig. 9**A). We usually recommend using 2 clips at the proximal side of the vessel, and an energy device to seal the distal side and divide the vessel (**Fig. 9**B). Because the specimen is usually manipulated in different directions, avoiding a clip on the distal stump reduces the risk of an accidental clip dislodgement and of a distal clip being included in the staple line during and subsequent stapling of the fissure. Although a new generation of clips has been designed with a nonslip system, it remains important to make a meticulous dissection of the vessel prior clip insertion (see Video 4). In expert hands, we have also the possibility to tie these vessels and use the energy device for distal division (**Fig. 9**C)

In case of central tumors or endobronchial lesions where there is not enough space for placing the stapler, the bronchus could be cut upstream of the tumor by a scalpel at a site free of tumor tissue. Then the bronchial stump can readily be closed by stapler by holding and pulling the sides by 2 traction stitches.

At the end of the operation, the surgical specimen is removed inside a specimen delivery bag designed for endoscopic surgery use, and that is then pulled out through the wound with a vigorous but gentle circular movement. When the tumor is not too big, we can use a simple surgical glove to lower costs. However, edges of the mouth of the glove must be grasped with long ring forceps to keep the mouth opened as the specimen is delivered into the glove.

For larger tumors, the limiting step preventing specimen retrieval is often the narrowness of the intercostal space, not the length of the skin incision (which is slightly elastic). A simple technique of cutting a rib anteriorly allows the intercostal space to open up without forceful rib spreading for large specimen retrieval.[14] The cut rib can be reapproximated using a double suture.

Right Upper Lobectomy

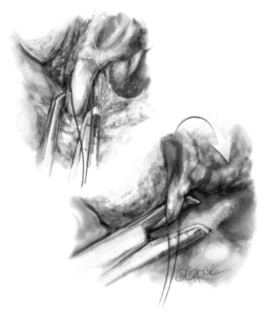

Fig. 8. The "rotation trick" to divide the right upper lobe vein by using a reticulated and curved tip stapler.

A right upper lobectomy procedure is ideal to showcase the tips and tricks of doing a uniportal

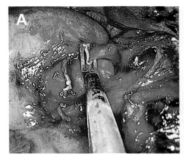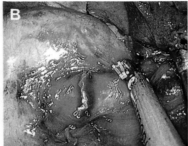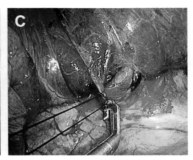

Fig. 9. (*A*) The use of a 45° applier to place a polymer clip on the base of the posterior ascending artery during a left upper lobectomy. (*B*) The energy device is used for distal division of this branch. (*C*) The V3 is tied by using a thoracoscopic knot pusher during an anterior right upper segmentectomy.

lobectomy. One must be aware of anatomic variations of the A2 and A3 artery branches. In approximately 90% of patients, there is a single A2 ascending artery that arises from the interlobar artery, but sometimes two A2 ascending arteries are described. In 15% of individuals, there may not be an A2 ascending artery, and in this case the posterior segment is fed entirely from the truncus anterior. The A3 arises solely from the truncus anterior in the majority of cases, but an additional or alternative supply can also be seen from A2 ascending artery in 25% of individuals, or there may be an A3 ascending artery that arises from the interlobar artery below the anterior trunk in approximately 15% of cases. Sometimes there is a common trunk of A2 and A6, so a careful dissection must be performed to preserve the A6 branch.[15,16]

The principal steps for a standard right upper lobectomy are as follows.

1. Identification of the upper vein and truncus anterior (Boyden's trunk).
2. Dissection and division of the truncus anterior.
3. Identification of the middle lobe vein and then division of the upper vein.
4. Dissection and division of the upper bronchus (after checking inflation of the middle and lower lobe).
5. Identification and division of the A2.
6. Completion of the fissure.

Tips and tricks

- The first maneuver to expose the hilum is to grasp the S3 segment, and retract it posteriorly and inferiorly. The assistant holds this grasper and the surgeon uses the long, curved suction device to expose the artery and vein to start the dissection.
- The angulation and direction of the stapler for right upper lobe vein, artery, and bronchus follows the "rule of the flexed arms," and is

normally with the stapler anvil angulated to the left.
- It is sometimes helpful to sling the upper vein with a tape to pull and enlarge the space for stapler insertion.
- In case of an incomplete fissure, it is very important to identify the middle lobe vein to define to define the interlobar plane, and to be sure the venous drainage of middle lobe is preserved.
- In some cases, when even after division of the artery there is not a good angle to insert the stapler for the vein, we can follow with the dissection and division of bronchus and even the posterior ascending artery to allow more rotation of the lobe, before returning to divide the vein at the end.
- Before the dissection of the bronchus from anteriorly, it is recommended to first grasp the lung on segment 1 and pull it anteriorly and inferiorly to expose the posterior side of the bronchus. This allows the surgeon to dissect the pleura above the intermedius bronchus, identify the bronchial artery, and remove the lymph nodes to facilitate dissection subsequent of the bronchus and insertion of staplers from anteriorly.
- In the majority of cases, the division of the right upper bronchus before tackling the A2 makes further management of this artery easy and safer. This is the most dangerous branch during a right upper lobectomy and one of the most frequent reasons of conversion during uniportal VATS.
- Before stapling the fissure (fissureless technique), it is mandatory to expose the middle lobe artery and remove adhesions from the entire stump of right upper lobe vein. The latter must be dissected as proximal as possible to avoid it being included in the stapling line of the fissure (the location of the anvil of the stapler must be always above the

middle lobe and interlobar artery and below the right upper lobe vein stump).

Right Lower Lobectomy

A right lower lobectomy can be the most difficult lobe when the fissure is oblique and incomplete because the origin of the A6 artery can arise in a very high position. In 80% of patients, the right lower lobe artery gives off the posteriorly oriented artery to S6 at about the same level as the origin of middle lobe artery. However, in 20% of cases, the A6 arises as 2 or very rarely 3 separate arteries from the lower lobe artery.[15,16]

When the interlobar fissure is complete, the artery is easily exposed within the fissure and dissected. In such patients, we can proceed in a sequence as follows.

1. Dissect the pulmonary ligament and identify the right lower and middle veins.
2. Dissect the anterior fissure between lower and middle lobes.
3. Complete dissection and division of the arterial branches for basal and A6 artery branches.
4. Dissect and divide the posterior part of the fissure.
5. Dissect and divide the lower lobe bronchus.

However, when the interlobar fissure is incomplete we have 2 options:

a. Lobectomy from bottom to top (fissureless technique): in this case dissect and divide the vein first, then bronchus, artery and finally fissure; or
b. Open the fissure from the hilum by identifying the lower and middle lobe vein from the hilum, and in a tunnel view expose the top of the bronchus and the artery, then finally place the anvil of the stapler above the surface of the artery and open the fissure (see **Fig. 7**).

Tips and tricks

- The right lower lobe must be retracted in a cephalad and lateral direction to expose the pulmonary ligament. We recommend cutting the posterior mediastinal pleura up to the bronchus, in this way better identification of the V6 vein branch is allowed.
- The stapler tip sometimes impacts against the spine as it is inserted around the vein, preventing it from fully passing the vein. Retraction of the lung forward and rotating the articulating stapler head clockwise (tip turned in a cephalad direction) allows the stapler to be passed parallel to the spine from caudal

to cephalad and avoid impacting onto the spine.

- When the origin of the A6 is higher that the origin of middle lobe artery, the best option is to dissect it and divide it separately, by using a stapler of by means of vascular clips (2 clips proximal and energy device distally).
- After the isolation of the right lower bronchus, while holding the lung laterally and anteriorly, place the stapler in a perpendicular way to the bronchus for cutting it.
- Once the A6 is identified, follow the dissection above the surface of the artery. The dissection of the posterior pleura exposes the bronchus intermedius and its bifurcation with right upper lobe bronchus, making the dissection of the posterior fissure easier from anterior side.
- It is important to remove all peribronchial lymph nodes, especially on the posterior side, and to dissect the bronchus as distal as possible.
- Always check inflation of the bronchus before firing the stapler to ensure that the middle lobe bronchus is preserved and patent.

Middle Lobectomy

The challenge with the right middle lobe is that the hilum is very close to the incision. In smaller patients, it is sometimes slightly more difficult to insert the entire head of the stapler to the hilar structures, and to maneuver instruments inside. The key is sometimes to manipulate the lung with the left hand holding the retractor, gently displacing it away from the single port to allow more room for insertion of the stapler or dissecting instruments with the right or dominant hand. In approximately one-half of patients, the A4 and A5 artery branches arise as separate branches from interlobar artery, but in another half they arise as common trunk before dividing. Less commonly, 3 separate branches are seen[15,16]

The main steps for a standard middle lobectomy are as follows.

1. Identification of the right lower and middle vein.
2. Dissection and division of the middle vein.
3. Dissection of the parenchyma and fissure between middle and lower lobes.
4. Dissection of the middle lobe bronchus and division with a stapler.
5. Identification and division of A4 and A5.
6. Division of the minor fissure between upper and middle lobe.

Tips and tricks

- Make the incision more anterior at the level of fifth intercostal space.

- Retract the middle lobe laterally and posteriorly for most of the operation, to allow the hilar structures to be approached from anteriorly.
- The use of curved tip staplers is very useful for division of middle lobe vein.
- Division of the anterior portion of the major fissure first allows more space for stapler insertion to divide the vein.
- After dividing the vein, the middle lobe bronchus is easily exposed. Be careful with the dissection to avoid damage of the artery behind. The suction device trick ensures a safe division of the bronchus (see Video 2).
- Once the bronchus is divided, do not apply too much traction to the lobe. The A4 and A5 branches can be divided between vascular clips applied with the 45° clip applier (proximal 2 clips and distal energy device).
- Once the vessels are divided, the last step is to divide the major fissure, and we must ensure that all distal stumps (artery, vein, and bronchus) are included in the resected middle lobe.

Right Pneumonectomy

To perform a right pneumonectomy by uniportal VATS we must first be totally sure that a lung-sparing procedure (such as a sleeve lobectomy) cannot be performed. It is always better to convert to an open sleeve procedure if possible than to persist with a VATS pneumonectomy.

Normally, a pneumonectomy is technically easier to perform than a lobectomy because no fissure needs to be managed. The only critical point of a VATS pneumonectomy is to achieve a short bronchial stump to reduce the risk of a bronchopleural fistula. In difficult cases, such as big tumors or cases after chemotherapy, intrapericardial control of the main pulmonary artery at the beginning of the operation is advised.

The principal steps for a standard right pneumonectomy are as follows.

1. Dissection of the upper, middle and lower veins.
2. Dissection and division of the main artery.
3. Division of the veins.
4. Dissection and division of the main bronchus.

Tips and tricks

- On the right side, the dissection and division of main pulmonary artery can be more difficult because the upper vein interferes with dissection. In that case, we recommend starting with vein division (rotation trick and suction device trick).

- If the common trunk of the artery is too short or is intrapericardial, there may not be enough space for placement of the stapler. In such cases, it is suggested to first identify and dissect the Boyden trunk to the upper lobe. This exposes more length on the right main pulmonary artery, allowing easier dissection and division.
- The direction of the stapler for dissection of the artery normally follows the rule of the flexed arms (anvil curved to the left).
- To divide the bronchus an endostapler can be used, but a transverse reticulated stapler (see **Fig. 12**) may be useful to achieve the shortest stump possible.
- For a bronchial stump at particular risk of a bronchopleural fistula (cases after chemoradiation, infected disease, etc) a flap must be used, such as from pleura, intercostal muscle, pericardial fat, or thymus tissue.

Left Upper Lobectomy

The same technique used with the right upper lobe is applied to dissect and divide the pulmonary vein and artery. Using the rotation trick (see **Fig. 8**) and/or the suction device trick as described (see **Fig. 5**), there is usually no problem first transecting the vein using an articulated stapler (see Video 1). On the left upper lobe, the variations of the anatomy are more frequent. Two to 7 artery branches may originate from the proximal left pulmonary artery to the upper lobe. It is important to also be aware of the possibility of a common left vein, which occurs in almost one-quarter of patients.[17,18]

The principal steps for a standard left upper lobectomy in a patient with a complete interlobar fissure could be as follows.

1. Dissection of the upper vein.
2. Identification, dissection, and division of the apical and anterior artery.
3. Division of the upper vein.
4. Identification and division of the lingular arteries.
5. Dissection of the anterior parenchyma and fissure.
6. Dissection of the posterior parenchyma and fissure (after identification of A6).
7. Dissection and division of the remaining arteries from the fissure.
8. Dissection and division of the upper bronchus.

The options for a left upper lobectomy with an incomplete interlobar fissure could be as follows.

a. Open the fissure as the first step. From a hilar view, create a tunnel between the upper and lower veins with identification of the bronchus and artery. The anvil of the stapler is placed over the artery, dividing the anterior portion of the fissure and allowing for the mobilization of the lobe (to allow the stapling of the vein from a different angle). Once the fissure is opened, we can follow the same steps as described.

b. We can perform the lobectomy from top to bottom as follows.

1. Dissection of the upper vein.
2. Identification, dissection, and division of the apical and anterior arteries.
3. Division of the upper vein.
4. Dissection and division of the upper bronchus with the suction device trick.
5. Dissection and division of lingular arteries and posterior ascending arteries.
6. Completion of the fissure (fissureless technique).

Tips and tricks

- If the distance between the upper vein and artery is enough we recommend dividing first the vein to easily expose the anterior artery (Video 1). The rotation trick and the suction device trick—coupled with the use of curved tip staplers—are extremely useful.
- In patients with no fissure, we must always expose both upper and lower lobe vein to avoid a catastrophic inadvertent division of a common vein.
- Dividing the vein first is helpful to provide more space in exposing and dissecting arterial branches behind, especially if dissection of the artery is difficult, such as in cases with severe lymphadenopathy.
- In the fissureless technique, the bronchus must be dissected with extreme caution using a right-angled clamp. The clamp must be kept in contact with the back wall of the bronchus at all times to prevent inadvertent puncture of the pulmonary artery behind it. Partial dissection or division of the anterior part of the fissure may often help to further improve exposure to the bronchus.
- The division of the first and second branches of the artery and of the upper vein allows for better lateral retraction of the left upper lobe laterally and hence better exposure of the left upper lobar bronchus. The suction device trick facilitates the insertion of the stapler and protects the lingular artery located just behind the bronchus (see **Fig. 6** and Video 2).
- Without the support of the bronchus, excessive force when dissection the small branches, lingular or posterior arteries can cause tearing and avulsion with major bleeding.

Left Lower Lobectomy

It is probably the easiest lobectomy when the interlobar fissure is complete, allowing easy access to the pulmonary artery. For performing a standard left lower lobectomy, proceed as follows.

1. Dissect the pulmonary ligament.
2. Identify and divide the lower lobe vein.
3. Dissect the anterior parenchyma and fissure.
4. Identify and divide the basal pyramid and A6 arterial branches.
5. Dissect the posterior parenchyma and fissure.
6. Dissect and divide the lower bronchus.

In case of an incomplete inter-lobar fissure, the same steps as for a right lower lobectomy with an incomplete fissure should be followed—with a bottom to top (fissureless) technique: ligament, vein, bronchus, artery and then fissure (Video 5).

Technical details

- The lingular artery must be always identified and preserved carefully in cases of partial or incomplete fissure, especially when using fissureless technique with a bottom to top sequence.
- When the origin of the lingular artery is very low, the A6 branch could be divided separately from the basal branches either by polymer clips (proximal 2 clips and distal energy device) or vascular stapler.
- After isolation of the left lower bronchus, and while holding the lung upward and anteriorly, place the stapler in a perpendicular way to the bronchus for transection to prevent a long stump.

Left Pneumonectomy

The most difficult part and the key point of left pneumonectomy is to cut the main bronchus close to the carina to get a shot stump and reduce the risk of postoperative bronchopleural fistula.

For performing a standard left pneumonectomy, proceed as follows.

1. Identify the upper and lower veins.
2. Identify and divide the main arteries.
3. Dissect and divide the upper vein and lower vein.
4. Divide the main bronchus.

Tips and tricks

- In case of difficulty in identification of the common trunk of the artery (because of severe lymphadenopathy or a very short trunk), open the pericardium and sling the artery intrapericardially. The same procedure could be done for dissection of the veins.
- We recommend opening and closing the stapler 2 times before firing the main pulmonary artery. This gentle precompression of the large artery may promote better staple formation and reduce oozing from the staple line after firing.
- In case of any need to protect the bronchial stump with a flap, the intercostal muscle of the same intercostal space as the uniport incision can be harvested and prepared under endoscopic vision.
- As described, it is very important to dissect the bronchus as proximal as possible to obtain a short stump. In doing so, extra care must be taken to avoid damage of recurrent laryngeal nerve under the aortic arch.
- The use of a transverse (eg, transverse reticulated) stapler is recommended to achieve a short stump. Once the stapler is closed, the bronchus is gently pulled toward the surgeon before firing to prevent the tip of the scalpel accidentally catching on adjacent tissue and causing an accident (**Fig. 10**; see Video 6).

Anatomic Segmentectomies

The way to approach the segments does not differ much from conventional VATS. Because the segmental vessels and bronchi are more distal and lateral, the angles for dissection and insertion of staplers are actually less limited (the more hilar or proximal the dissection, the more difficulty to insert staplers).[19],[20] In most segmentectomies, small segmental or subsegmental vessels can be secured by using clips or ligatures before dividing (staplers not required). The 45° polymer clip applicators are extremely useful and safe for segmental vessels. It should be noted that the more distal the bronchovascular anatomy, the more likely it is to find anatomic variants. It is always recommended to ventilate the lung before cutting the segmental bronchus. The boundary between inflated and noninflated lung will serve as a good guide to delimit the intersegmental plane[21] (see Video 7).

Lymphadenectomy

The concept of advanced instrumentation is ideal for lymph node dissection, and the idea is to avoid grasping the lymph nodes during a complete resection[6] (see Video 8). Thanks to a high-definition view, the long curved instruments specifically designed for uniportal VATS, and modern energy devices, the uniportal technique is an excellent approach to accomplish a complete lymph node dissection.[22]

For right paratracheal (#4R) dissection, the anti-Trendelenburg position is very helpful, making the lung "fall down" caudally. We recommend starting the dissection from below the azygos by opening the space between the cava, artery, and right main bronchus. The long, curved suction device should be used to retract the vena cava or the azygos vein to better expose the plane (**Fig. 11**A). The use of an energy device, hook, or lymph node grasper is useful for lymph node dissection in this area. Once the package of lymph nodes is freed from below the azygous vein, the pleura above the azygos vein is opened in a triangular window delineated by the vena cava, azygos vein, and trachea. Then, the package of lymph nodes can be pulled up above the azygos vein and retracted by the long curved suction device, and the dissection is continued to remove the whole package en bloc (**Fig. 11**B). It is important

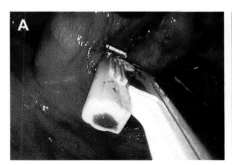
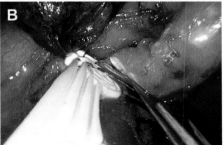

Fig. 10. Transection of the left upper lobe bronchus using a conventional transverse reticulated stapler. (*A*) The anvil of the stapler is inserted behind the main bronchus and closed as proximal as possible. (*B*) The bronchus is pulled toward the surgeon and the bronchus is incised by using a long scalpel.

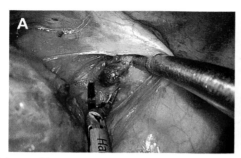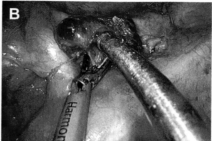

Fig. 11. Advanced instrumentation during paratracheal lymph node dissection below the azygos vein (*A*) and above the azygos vein (*B*).

to always identify the vagus nerve to avoid iatrogenic damage.

For subcarinal dissection, using the Trendelenburg position with an anterior table rotation facilitates the exposure. Preliminary division of the pulmonary ligament provides better access to the subcarinal space. It is recommended to use a sponge stick to compress the posterior part of the lung or a grasper to pull it anteriorly toward the surgeon. The assistant must hold a camera and the grasper with the other hand in the upper part of the incision and the surgeon must work with manual instrumentation below the camera and grasper. The vagus nerve (running between the carina and the esophagus) must be preserved. On the left side, it is possible to encircle the inferior pulmonary vein with a tape and pull to increase the exposure of the subcarinal area. The dissection must follow the inferior part of ipsilateral main bronchus past the carina, and expose the contralateral main bronchus to ensure that the real subcarinal space has been reached. Special care must be taken to avoid damage of the esophagus and contralateral bronchus.

Advanced Cases

In cases where a sleeve resection is required, it is important to fully release the pulmonary ligament and perform a subcarinal lymphadenectomy before starting the suturing.[23] This is to give more mobility to the airway ends to be sutured together, and hence reduce tension on the anastomosis. The anastomosis is usually performed with a 3/0 PDS or Prolene continuous suture with a wire fitted with 2 needles, knotting once on the anterior side after completing both sides of the bronchial circumference (**Fig. 12**A).[8,24,25]

For tumors involving the trachea or carina, high-frequency jet ventilation can be used, thus not interfering with the anastomosis (**Fig. 12**B and Video 9). However, we must always have ready an intrafield intubation system in case of need.[6]

When the pulmonary artery may be compromised (calcified adenopathies or tumors invading the artery), it is best to expose and control the main artery (by encircling and/or clamping) before dissection[26] (see Video 10). In case of bleeding, this provides more control over the situation and allow rescue with more safely. The safest method is to clamp the main artery as proximal as possible. The safest form of clamping is with a vascular clamp (**Fig. 12**C), although a tourniquet or even a bulldog clamp may also be used (**Fig. 12**D). Intrapericardial dissection of the pulmonary artery gives a wider and more secure margin of clamping. A proximal clamp below the ductus arteriosus on the left side also serves as an anchorage system to avoid accidental displacement if a tourniquet system is used. It is very important to perform careful and meticulous instrumentation once the clamp is placed, to avoid any kind of displacement of the clamp. If we use a thoracoscopic clamp, it should be placed in the inferior part of the incision to reduce the risk of inadvertent displacement.[27] In case of vascular reconstruction, it is necessary to clamp either the inferior pulmonary vein or the basal trunk of the pulmonary artery for proximal control.[28] In this case, the use of a bulldog clamp or a tourniquet is most recommended, and the latter can be pulled and fixed with a polymer vascular clip to maintain the compression (see **Fig. 12**D).

When a vascular sleeve resection is needed, the end-to-end vascular anastomosis can be performed with a running monofilament suture (Prolene 4 or 5/0, one thread with 2 needles) in 2 steps: the first suture line must be at the posterior wall of the anastomosis from a back to front direction using one of the needles, and then the other needle is used for a running suture to complete the anastomosis of the anterior wall (see **Fig. 12**C). Both ends are tied together at the anterior side.[29]

Once the vascular suture is completed, the distal clamp is removed to allow de-airing by the

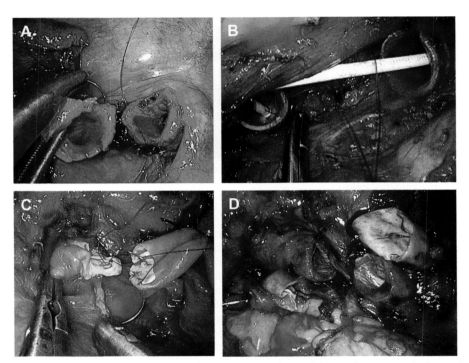

Fig. 12. Surgical image showing the technique for sleeve procedures. (*A*) Running suture during a right upper lobe sleeve anastomosis. (*B*) Use of a high-frequency ventilation jet during a right side carinal sleeve resection. (*C*) Running suture for sleeve vascular anastomosis using a proximal thoracoscopic clamp and distal tourniquet to control the pulmonary artery. (*D*) Proximal and distal control of the left pulmonary artery with a tourniquet during a double sleeve procedure.

return flow of blood, and the suture is tied once the artery is filled. The proximal clamp is released very slowly, observing for intactness of the anastomosis. In case of a double bronchial and vascular sleeve resection, the bronchial anastomosis should be performed first to reduce excessive tension on the vascular suture line.[29]

Unisurgeon Uniportal Video-assisted Thoracoscopic Surgery

One of the latest advances in uniportal VATS is the possibility of using a robotic articulated arm that holds the camera stable. There are several available systems of articulated arms, such as one where the surgeon manually moves a pneumatic arm, and one where the arm is voice controlled. This technology potentially obviates the need for an assistant altogether, and in the hands of very experienced uniportal VATS surgeons this enables a unisurgeon, assistant-free operation.

This approach requires that the surgeon must learn to handle several instruments with 1 hand and to be able to exert the same bimanual instrumentation. It is mandatory to learn "double finger instrumentation," which means that with 1 hand (usually the left hand) 2 instruments are held and moved at the same time, a retractor to grasp the lung and provide exposure with 2 digits, and a long curved suction to perform the tasks as described with the remaining digits (**Fig. 13**). The right hand is used to wield the energy device or a dissector instrument as described. Sometimes, it is very helpful to support the ring clamp or grasper on a part of the articulated arm to release a hand to wield another instrument (see Video 11).

With conventional or uniportal VATS with an assistant, the camera is constantly adjusted to actively maintain the zone of dissection in the middle of the screen. However, with a unisurgeon approach, it is the reverse: the camera is fixed and the surgeon must constantly adjust the retraction of the lung to position the dissection zone in the center of the screen (see Video 7).

There are some advantages to not having an assistant scrubbed in. First, an assistant often fatigues during an operation, leading to worsening camera handling and retraction as the operation progresses. The unisurgeon approach may avoid this. Second, without an assistant standing right at the surgeon's elbow, the surgeon has more room to work comfortably on that side of the

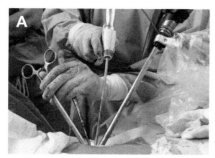
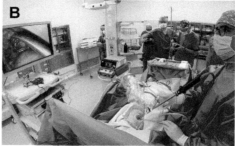

Fig. 13. Unisurgeon uniportal video-assisted thoracoscopic surgery photo showing the technique during a right lower lobectomy with the help of an articulated arm and no assistant. (*A*) The "double finger technique" handling 2 instruments with the left hand. (*B*) Position of surgeon and the camera.

operating table, and a greater range of arm movements is possible without interference during the instrumentation. However, an assistant should always be available to be called in to help in case of bleeding or other on-table complications.

SUMMARY

The learning of technical details on uniportal VATS is essential to perform a safe, quick, and oncologically sound anatomic resection. Small details make big differences in uniportal VATS. However, the uniportal technique has evolved during the last few years to become almost an entirely new concept: "advanced uniportal VATS." This development emphasizes performing surgery with the least number of devices possible, reducing the crowding of multiple instruments via the single intercostal space.

We must keep in mind that uniportal is distinct from other forms of minimally invasive thoracic surgery, and the technique of exposure and stapler insertion is totally different. Despite the learning curve for uniportal VATS being short, experience with conventional VATS alone is not enough to ensure full proficiency with uniportal VATS. Surgeons experienced with a 2-port technique or with anterior thoracotomy approach will probably adopt the uniportal concept faster than those experienced with 3 ports only. However, ultimately mastering the uniportal VATS technique requires visiting experienced high-volume uniportal VATS centers, and attending training courses with hands-on wet labs run by the experts.[30]

SUPPLEMENTARY DATA

Supplementary data related to this article can be found online at 10.1016/j.thorsurg.2017.06.004.

REFERENCES

1. Gonzalez D, Paradela M, Garcia J, et al. Single-port video-assisted thoracoscopic lobectomy. Interact Cardiovasc Thorac Surg 2011;12:514–5.
2. Ng CS, Lau KK, González-Rivas D, et al. Evolution in surgical approach and techniques for lung cancer. Thorax 2013;68:681.
3. Rocco G, Martucci N, La Manna C, et al. Ten-year experience on 644 patients undergoing single-port (uniportal) video-assisted thoracoscopic surgery. Ann Thorac Surg 2013;96:434–8.
4. Wang BY, Liu CY, Hsu PK, et al. Single-incision versus multiple-incision thoracoscopic lobectomy and segmentectomy: a propensity-matched analysis. Ann Surg 2015;261:793–9.
5. Sihoe ADL. The evolution of VATS lobectomy. In: Cardoso P, editor. Topics in thoracic surgery. Croatia (Rijeka): Intech; 2011. p. 181–210.
6. Gonzalez-Rivas D, Yang Y, Calvin NG. Advances in uniportal video-assisted thoracoscopic surgery: pushing the envelope. Thorac Surg Clin 2016; 26(2):187–201.
7. Gonzalez-Rivas D, Paradela M, Fernandez R, et al. Uniportal video-assisted thoracoscopic lobectomy: two years of experience. Ann Thorac Surg 2013; 95:426–32.
8. Gonzalez-Rivas D, Yang Y, Sekhniaidze D, et al. Uniportal video-assisted thoracoscopic bronchoplastic and carinal sleeve procedures. J Thorac Dis 2016; 8:S210–22.
9. Hirai K, Takeuchi S, Usuda J. Single-incision thoracoscopic surgery and conventional video-assisted thoracoscopic surgery: a retrospective comparative study of perioperative clinical outcomes. Eur J Cardiothorac Surg 2015;49(Suppl 1):i37–41.
10. Sihoe ADL. The evolution of minimally invasive thoracic surgery: implications for the practice of uniportal thoracoscopic surgery. J Thorac Dis 2014;6: S604–17.
11. Gonzalez-Rivas D, Fernandez R, de la Torre M, et al. Thoracoscopic lobectomy through a single incision.

Multimed Man Cardiothorac Surg 2012;2012: mms007.

12. Wang H, Zhou X, Xie D, et al. Uniportal video-assisted thoracic surgery—the experiences of Shanghai Pulmonary Hospital. J Vis Surg 2016;2:56.

13. Sihoe DLA. Uniportal videoassisted thoracic surgery (VATS) lobectomy. Ann Cardiothorac Surg 2016;5: 133–44.

14. Sihoe AD, Chawla S, Paul S, et al. Technique for delivering large tumors in video-assisted thoracoscopic lobectomy. Asian Cardiovasc Thorac Ann 2014;22:319–28.

15. Pearson FG, Cooper JD, Deslauriers J, et al. Anatomy of the lung. Thoracic surgery. 2nd edition. Philadelphia: Churchill Livingstone; 2002. p. 427–41.

16. Shields TW, LoCicero J, Ponn RB, et al. Surgical anatomy of the lungs. General thoracic surgery. 6th edition. Philadelphia: Lippincott Williams & Wilkins; 2005. p. 59–73.

17. Healey JE Jr. An anatomic survey of anomalous pulmonary veins: their clinical significance. J Thorac Surg 1952;23:433–44.

18. Irene A, Theodoros K, Konstantinos N. Pulmonary vein anatomical variation during videothoracoscopy-assisted surgical lobectomy. Surg Radiol Anat 2016; 39(2):229–31.

19. Gonzalez-Rivas D, Mendez L, Delgado M, et al. Uniportal video-assisted thoracoscopic anatomic segmentectomy. J Thorac Dis 2013;5(Suppl 3): S226–33.

20. Gonzalez-Rivas D. Single incision video-assisted thoracoscopic anatomic segmentectomy. Ann Cardiothorac Surg 2014;3(2):204–7.

21. Watanabe A, Ohori S, Nakashima S, et al. Feasibility of video-assisted thoracoscopic surgery segmentectomy for selected peripheral lung carcinomas. Eur J Cardiothorac Surg 2009;35:775–80.

22. Guerrero WG, Gonzalez-Rivas D, Hernandez-Arenas LA, et al. Techniques and difficulties dealing with hilar and interlobar benign lymphadenopathy in uniportal VATS. J Vis Surg 2016;2:23.

23. Gonzalez-Rivas D, Fernandez R, Fieira E, et al. Uniportal video-assisted thoracoscopic bronchial sleeve lobectomy: first report. J Thorac Cardiovasc Surg 2013;145(6):1676–7.

24. Gonzalez-Rivas D, Yang Y, Stupnik T, et al. Uniportal video-assisted thoracoscopic bronchovascular, tracheal and carinal resections. Eur J Cardiothorac Surg 2015;49(Suppl 1):i6–16.

25. Gonzalez-Rivas D, Sihoe AD. Uniportal video-assisted thoracoscopic lobectomy. Shields, in press.

26. Gonzalez-Rivas D, Fieira E, Delgado M, et al. Uniportal video-assisted thoracoscopic sleeve lobectomy and other complex resections. J Thorac Dis 2014;6(S6):674–81.

27. Gonzalez-Rivas D, Delgado M, Fieira E, et al. Double sleeve uniportal video-assisted thoracoscopic lobectomy for non-small cell lung cancer. Ann Cardiothorac Surg 2014;3(2):E2.

28. Gonzalez-Rivas D, Delgado M, Fieira E, et al. Single-port video-assisted thoracoscopic lobectomy with pulmonary artery reconstruction. Interact Cardiovasc Thorac Surg 2013;17:889–91.

29. Huang J, Li J, Qiu Y, et al. Thoracoscopic double sleeve lobectomy in 13 patients: a series report from multi-centers. J Thorac Dis 2015;7(5): 834–42.

30. Sihoe AD. Opportunities and challenges for thoracic surgery collaborations in China: a commentary. J Thorac Dis 2016;8:S414–26.

Are There Contraindications for Uniportal Video-Assisted Thoracic Surgery?

Alan D.L. Sihoe, MBBChir, MA(Cantab), FRCSEd(CTh), FCSHK, FHKAM, FCCP[a,b,c,*]

KEYWORDS

- Video-assisted thoracic surgery (VATS) • Uniportal • Safety • Contraindications • Evidence

KEY POINTS

- Allowing oneself to indulge in illusory superiority when it comes to uniportal video-assisted thoracic surgery (VATS) can harm patients and the specialty.
- One must be clear about the absolute and relative contraindications for VATS: those conditions that should deter from even attempting a uniportal approach.
- Once the operation is started, one must also bear in mind those situations that should prompt one to stop persisting with uniportal VATS and convert.
- Only by first safeguarding patients in this way can the aspiring uniportal VATS surgeon go on to safely master the approach and explore its benefits.

SO YOU THINK YOU ARE A GREAT SURGEON?

In a classic study, 93% of surveyed drivers in the United States deemed themselves to be above average in terms of driving skills, and 88% felt their driving safety was also above average.[1] This echoed an earlier study by the United States College Board, which found that 70% of students felt they were above average in terms of leadership skills, and 85% felt they were above average in terms of being able to get along with others, including 25% who placed themselves in the top 1% in this ability.[2]

Such studies often elicit laughter. However, there is no reason to believe that surgeons are immune to this well-recognized phenomenon of "illusory superiority."[3] For surgeons reading this article, simply ask yourself: Have you never felt that your own skills are superior to your colleagues? The culture of surgery is inherently geared toward generating practitioners of great self-confidence, which may even exceed one's concern for patients.[4]

Today, as worldwide interest in uniportal video-assisted thoracic surgery (VATS) grows,[5–8] it is inevitable that increasing numbers of thoracic surgeons are rushing to learn this technique.[8–11] In this scenario, illusory superiority may blind many aspiring surgeons to the reality that not every surgeon or every center is suited to perform it. Instead, illusory overestimation of one's own surgical prowess, coupled with spectacular reports of complex surgery being feasible with uniportal VATS,[12,13] may easily lead one to believe that it is "easy."

The unfortunate consequences of this are 2-fold. First, in the early days of VATS in the

[a] Department of Surgery, The University of Hong Kong, Hong Kong, China; [b] The University of Hong Kong Shenzhen Hospital, Shenzhen, China; [c] Department of Thoracic Surgery, Tongji University, Shanghai Pulmonary Hospital, Shanghai, China
* Department of Surgery, Li Ka Shing Faculty of Medicine, The University of Hong Kong, Hong Kong, China.
E-mail address: adls1@hku.hk

Thorac Surg Clin 27 (2017) 373–380
http://dx.doi.org/10.1016/j.thorsurg.2017.06.005
1547-4127/17/© 2017 Elsevier Inc. All rights reserved.

1990s, many were also eager to jump on the bandwagon of this exciting new approach and publish their own results.[14] However, some studies reported negative results, which set back the adaptation of VATS for many years.[15–17] It was only gradually realized that not all those reporting their results were performing proper or "complete" VATS,[18] and that failure to do so could compromise patient outcomes.[19,20] In layman terms, some "bad drivers" were possibly tainting the track record of the "good drivers" by having their results counted among the latter's. Unless training is well-regulated, there is a risk that poor results from those performing uniportal incorrectly may taint the track record of the approach as a whole and set its development back for years.[11]

The second potential consequence from about illusory superiority goes much deeper than this. If surgeons attempt operations that they or their units are not suited to perform, patients' lives are potentially put at risk. One very regrettable mishap in 2015 that was widely reported occurred during a live surgery demonstration, when reportedly the surgical team persisted with a highly difficulty laparoscopic procedure despite significant intraoperative problems being encountered.[21] Whether the failure to convert to an open procedure (despite apparent calls for this from the audience) was owing to the illusory superiority of the team is not known. What is known is that the patient died. There is a clearly need to protect patients by defining limits on how far a surgeon should push him or herself in pursuing a particular technique. In other words, for an approach like uniportal VATS, it is necessary to be aware of the contraindications.

REASONS NOT TO PERFORM UNIPORTAL VIDEO-ASSISTED THORACIC SURGERY

A *contraindication* is defined in the Merriam-Webster Dictionary as "something (as a symptom or condition) that makes a particular treatment or procedure inadvisable."[22] In this context, it is first necessary to point out that lack of evidence saying that a surgical approach should always be used should not be misconstrued as an absolute dictum saying it should never be used. Evidence that an approach is harmful is a contraindication, but lack of evidence that it is beneficial is not.

This author previously published a systematic review in 2016 summarizing the evidence for and against the use of the uniportal VATS approach for lobectomy.[11] Given that there had only been a few years since uniportal VATS lobectomy was first performed,[6] it was not surprising that relatively few clinical data had been collected. Only a

handful of studies comparing the postoperative outcomes for uniportal VATS with those of conventional VATS had been published.[23–30] From those studies, only limited conclusions could be drawn about the supposed benefits of uniportal VATS:

i. *Operation:* Only 2 of the 7 studies providing data in this area found that uniportal VATS gave shorter operation times, less blood loss, and higher yields from lymph node dissection.[25,27] However, the absolute differences were small and both of these studies came from the same center. Another study actually showed that operation times were longer with uniportal VATS.[26] The remaining 4 studies found no difference between the approaches in terms of intraoperative parameters.

ii. *Pain and Morbidity:* Only 2 studies found that uniportal VATS gave lower postoperative pain, and only 1 associated it with quicker cessation of analgesic use and a lesser incidence of paresthesia.[26,28] None of the studies found that overall morbidity rates were lower among uniportal patients.

iii. *Recovery:* Only 1 study found that uniportal VATS gave shorter postoperative duration of stay,[27] but another study found that postoperative stay was longer after uniportal VATS.[30] The remaining studies found no difference between the approaches in terms of chest drain durations or durations of stay.

It would, thus, be fair to say that the evidence to support the use of the uniportal VATS approach over conventional VATS for all lobectomy operations ranges from weak to nonexistent. In terms of cancer survival after uniportal VATS lobectomy, there have been no large studies at all in this regard. There is simply not enough evidence to say that uniportal VATS should be done as the approach of choice. However, the volume of case series that have demonstrated the safety and feasibility of uniportal VATS in a large variety of clinical situations is large.[7,8,12,13,22–29] It can be argued that there is adequate evidence to say that uniportal VATS can be done.[11]

The lack of evidence in support of uniportal VATS in itself is not evidence to not perform it. Rather, now that it has been demonstrated to be feasible, this lack of comparative data should be a call for surgeons to explore the approach and create more data that will define its role in modern thoracic surgery. However, to safeguard patients as discussed, rules and contraindications should be established whilst that exploration is conducted.

CONTRAINDICATIONS: ARE THERE ANY?

The next distinction to note is that between a contraindication for uniportal VATS and an indication for conversion. A contraindication for a surgical approach may be regarded as a reason not to commence that approach, usually because it carries a risk of harm that outweighs the chance of benefit. An indication for conversion should be regarded as a reason not to persist with that approach. In this case, there may not have been any contraindications to begin with preoperatively, but the evolving clinical picture during the surgery may suggest that to carry on would entail a risk of harm outweighing the benefit.

In terms of contraindications for uniportal VATS, reference should first be made to the history of conventional VATS.[14] In the early days of conventional VATS, a long list of contraindications existed for the approach.[31] These are summarized in **Table 1**. However, with increasing experience, most of the absolute contraindications in the early days have now shifted to the relative contraindications column. Nowadays, virtually no VATS surgeon would consider pleural adhesions a significant problem.[8,32] Previous surgery and other sources of intrathoracic adhesions are also readily dealt with.[33] For fused fissures, a fissure-less technique is now standard practice for many VATS surgeons.[8,14,34] For large tumors, these can be delivered even via relatively small VATS wounds using a simple rib-cutting technique.[35] Sleeve resections are also possible by VATS, both bronchial and vascular.[36,37] Even the traditional requirement for good single-lung ventilation is presently being circumvented by the marriage of nonintubated anesthetic techniques with VATS.[38]

However, the one remaining absolute contraindication to conventional VATS is still the most important. That is, if the surgeon and his or her team are not completely trained, equipped, and comfortable with any VATS procedure, it should not be done. Even if reports exist for the use of VATS in all of these situations, any doubt in the team's ability to safely complete a VATS procedure should automatically make that VATS procedure 'inadvisable,' and that is the definition of a contraindication. There should be no excuse for using any patient as a training tool. This is especially true given that opportunities are so readily available for training in VATS nowadays should anyone feel uncomfortable with VATS.[10,39] There is, of course, the possibility that a surgical team is unaware that the limits of safety are being exceeded when VATS is being contemplated over other management strategies, again a situation of illusory superiority. One cure for this is to always use a multidisciplinary team approach to managing all patients with thoracic malignancy, where other specialties may be able to offer reasonable alternative strategies.[40,41]

These lessons from conventional VATS all apply to uniportal VATS. The same difficult situations in thoracic surgery that are relative contraindications

Table 1
A summary of the absolute and relative contraindications for conventional (multiportal) VATS lobectomy: the early days of VATS versus today

	Absolute Contraindications	Relative Contraindications
Early days of VATS	• Surgeon or team unprepared • Pleural adhesions • Previous surgery or pleurodesis • Previous hilar irradiation • Calcified lymph nodes • Fused interlobar fissures • Large tumors (>4 cm) • Tracheobronchial reconstructions • Cannot tolerate single-lung ventilation	
VATS today	• Surgeon or team unprepared	• Pleural adhesions • Previous surgery or pleurodesis • Previous hilar irradiation • Calcified lymph nodes • Fused interlobar fissures • Large tumors (>4 cm) • Tracheobronchial reconstructions • Cannot tolerate single-lung ventilation

Abbreviation: VATS, video-assisted thoracic surgery.

for conventional VATS may also be regarded as relative contraindications for uniportal VATS (see **Table 1**). Namely, adhesions, fused fissures, calcified lymph nodes, and large tumors are readily dealt with by experienced uniportal VATS surgeons.[8,42] Complex sleeve resections have also been reported by the most experienced uniportal VATS surgeons.[12,43] Uniportal VATS has furthermore been shown to be compatible with nonintubated anesthesia in the most experienced units.[44,45]

Nevertheless, it cannot be emphasized enough that these situations are relative contraindications only in the most experienced centers with the most experienced surgeons. The absolute contraindication for conventional VATS remains an absolute contraindication for uniportal VATS. For any surgeon not completely trained, equipped, and comfortable with any uniportal VATS procedure, those relative contraindications must immediately be considered as absolute contraindications. Illusory superiority in each surgeon anxious to practice this exciting new uniportal VATS approach must be balanced by seeking adequate training, a multidisciplinary team approach to management, and common sense.

This still begs the question: How does a surgeon—or a patient—know if he or she is ready to perform a particular uniportal procedure. Unfortunately, there is as yet no established system of credentialing for conventional—let alone uniportal—VATS. The Society of Thoracic Surgeons in the United States has issued an expert consensus statement, neatly summarizing criteria by which surgeons and institutes beginning a new thoracic surgical technique may be assessed and credentialed.[46] A handful of professional societies have also implemented structured programs for systematic training in VATS.[39] However, a universally recognized system or set of standards for credentialing in uniportal VATS remains a long way away. Until then, it behooves surgeons to maintain self-discipline and conscientiousness to avoid commencing any uniportal VATS procedure for which he or she is ill-prepared.

CONVERSION: THE PATIENT'S LAST LINE OF DEFENSE

As discussed, the literature suggests few absolute contraindications to uniportal VATS in experienced hands—but this can be easily misconstrued by those with inadequate experience to mean they have license to try uniportal surgery on any patient. Once a surgeon embarks on a given surgical approach like this, the last line of defense for the patient is conversion in the event of any intraoperative problem.

Uniportal VATS is without doubt a product of an incremental evolution of VATS, which itself carries the same basic principles as traditional open surgery.[8,14] Should any complications arise during uniportal VATS, it is important for the surgeon to fall back to an approach with which he or she is familiar so that the complication can be managed safely. This can be falling back just a step or two to 2-port or 3-port VATS, or all the way back to a full open thoracotomy. This is quite a standard teaching in most papers teaching uniportal VATS.[8,42]

However, for this simple message of 'convert when you are in trouble' to work, there are 2 prerequisites. The first is that the surgeon has enough experience with conventional VATS and/or open surgery to handle the complication once conversion has been done. If the surgeon (or his or her supervisor) does not have this experience, this should be an absolute contraindication for uniportal VATS as described. In this case, the surgeon and the team is advised to master the earlier steps along the VATS evolution pathway before proceeding to uniportal VATS.[8] Second, the surgeon must be able to recognize those situations when conversion is necessary. The lesson of the mishap during live surgery teaches that self-awareness must be maintained during surgery to avoid missing those indications for conversion. To facilitate this, the author suggests a simple system of "ABCD" categorizing these indications (from most to least absolute).

Anesthetic

Although it is suggested that nonintubated anesthesia has been demonstrated to be feasible, it is currently available in only a handful of centers.[38,44,45] For most uniportal VATS operations in most centers around the world, achieving good single-lung ventilation remains essential. Without good ipsilateral lung collapse during surgery, the operation becomes virtually impossible because of lack of space within the chest to work. Under such circumstances, it is quicker and safer to convert to either conventional VATS (where the extra ports allow better retraction of the lung) or open thoracotomy.

Bleeding

When major bleeding occurs during uniportal VATS (or conventional VATS for that matter), the mantra is another ABC: apply, breathe, and consider. The first instinct must always be to apply pressure to the site of bleeding. This can be done with a sucker, a peanut pledget, or a sponge stick.[8,47] Bleeding can be more rapid than at first realized, and unless pressure is applied very promptly the total blood loss can accumulate surprisingly rapidly. This can then compromise subsequent remedial action if the patient is already suffering from volume loss and tending toward shock. It is, therefore, essential for the surgeon and the team to develop the instinct to apply pressure immediately no matter how 'small' the bleeding seems to be at first, and to always have a pledget and/or sponge stick available for this before starting each VATS procedure.

Once the hemorrhaging is slowed or stopped temporarily by the pressure, it is essential for the surgeon to pause and breathe. This second step is not passively doing nothing. Instead, it is an active step requiring the surgeon (and the team) to calm himself or herself down. In many cases of bad outcomes after bleeding, the initial bleeding is not catastrophic, but it is the panic on the part of the surgeon that may worsen the situation to a dangerous level.[48] In an anxious rush to try to stop the bleeding, a surgeon may make ill-considered attempts to suture (which can enlarge some bleeding sites) or clip (which blocks subsequent attempts to repair), and so on. The breathe step is necessary to calm not only oneself, but the whole team. It is the opportunity to ensure everyone—from assistants, to anesthetists, to nurses—understands clearly what has happened and what needs to be done next. Help may also be called in from other surgeons of the team or even from other surgical specialties as appropriate.

The third step is to consider whether conversion to thoracotomy is necessary. The first consideration is. "What is the damage?" If the bleeding site is small enough to suture, or an avulsed vessel still has enough proximal length to be clipped safely, then a surgeon with adequate VATS experience may wish to attempt a VATS repair. However, a big hole on a major vessel may prompt conversion sooner rather than later. The next consideration is, "How much of the operation has been done?" If the bleeding has occurred late in the operation when it is almost finished, it may be possible to complete the operation promptly without converting. However, if the operation has only just started, and persisting with VATS would mean a protracted struggle while there is an continuing risk of ongoing bleeding, then it may be more prudent to convert. The final consideration is, "Do I have what I need to control the bleeding?" This involves whether one has the required experience and skills, the right equipment (such as effective hemostats, instruments, etc),

and an adequately competent team. The latter is especially important. If the assistant is not capable of maintaining clear visualization with the video-thoracoscope or help with the retraction, or if the nursing staff cannot understand and support what one is trying to do, then even the simplest VATS attempt at bleeding control can quickly spiral out of control. In such situations, it is also best to convert without hesitation.

Cancer Related (or Pathology Related)

During an operation, a surgeon may find that the pathology may be more advanced than anticipated. The decision of whether or not conversion is necessary then becomes a matter of assessing one's own experience. For example, unexpected proximal extension of a tumor may be dealt with by uniportal VATS if one has the experience.[12,43] Unexpected mediastinal nodal metastases may be dealt with by VATS if one has the necessary skills for a good nodal clearance by VATS.[49,50] Even when performing surgery for complex sequestration, the appearance of unexpected anomalous feeding vessels can also be readily handled using uniportal VATS, if one is experienced.[51] However, once again, the surgeon must be called on to judge carefully whether he or she truly has the ability to persist with VATS. Any doubt should prompt consideration of conversion. A lung cancer patient will fare better with an R0 resection after conversion to thoracotomy than he or she would after a uniportal procedure that only gives an R1/2 resection.

Difficult Situations

As noted, difficult elements such as pleural adhesions, fused fissures, and large tumors are no longer regarded as serious contraindications by experienced VATS surgeons.[34,35,42] Calcified lymph nodes remain one of the more common reasons for converting from VATS to open surgery,[32,52] but even so the absolute incidence of conversions because of calcified nodes is not high and the conversion itself does not harm patients significantly. Compared with the cancer-related indications for conversion, these difficult situations perhaps do not prompt conversion as strongly because they are benign and do not affect patient treatment outcomes as substantially. It may be reasonable to persist longer with uniportal VATS when tackling these, and they represent a fair opportunity for surgeons to home their uniportal technique without compromising patient outcomes. Nevertheless, the surgeon is still cautioned not to get too carried away and end up excessively and needlessly prolonging surgery simply for the sake of persisting with uniportal VATS. There is an old saying: "The minute you think of giving up, think of the reason why you held on so long." In the case of uniportal VATS, as soon as one converts, one usually realizes that trying to persist was not worthwhile for the patient.

SUMMARY

In this special issue on uniportal VATS, virtually all the other articles extol the virtues of uniportal VATS and demonstrate how it can be used in a wide range of operations. The reader can easily—and understandably—be misled into thinking that (1) he or she must perform uniportal VATS, and (2) he or she can perform it easily. Neither belief is true. Regarding the first, the current evidence does not support the notion that uniportal VATS is superior to any other VATS approach, and hence readers should not feel under undue pressure to adopt this approach (at least until future evidence may prove otherwise). Regarding the second, readers need to be aware that there is undoubtedly a degree of publication bias when it comes to uniportal VATS. Authors tend only to submit papers reporting their prowess at uniportal VATS, but not their difficulties; and journals tend to publish articles claiming ever more complex and high-risk procedures can be done by this approach. Such bias can facilitate the misconception that the technique is not so challenging and that anyone can immediately do it without much preparation. That misconception is further aided by the human tendency toward illusory superiority: "If those authors can do it, why can't I?"

Because allowing oneself to indulge in illusory superiority when it comes to uniportal VATS can harm patients and the specialty, it is important for every VATS surgeon to remain vigilant. One must be clear about the absolute and relative contraindications for VATS: those conditions that should deter from even attempting a uniportal approach. Once the operation is started, one must also bear in mind those situations (ABCD) that should prompt one to stop persisting with uniportal VATS and convert. Only by first safeguarding patients in this way can the aspiring uniportal VATS surgeon go on to safely master the approach and explore its benefits.

REFERENCES

1. Svenson O. Are we all less risky and more skillful than our fellow drivers? (PDF). Acta Psychol 1981; 47:143–8.

2. Alicke MD, Govorun O. The better-than-average effect. In: Alicke MD, Dunning DA, Krueger JI, editors. The self in social judgment. Studies in self and identity. London: Psychology Press; 2005. p. 85–106. ISBN 978-1-84169-418-4. OCLC 58054791.

3. Hoorens V. Self-enhancement and superiority biases in social comparison. European review of social psychology, vol. 4(1). London: Psychology Press; 1993. p. 113–39.

4. Srivastava R. When medical hierarchy and surgeons' egos compete with patients' best interests. The Guardian. 2016. Available at: https://www.theguardian.com/commentisfree/2016/mar/28/when-medical-hierarchy-and-surgeons-egos-compete-with-patients-best-interests. Accessed February 6, 2017.

5. Rocco G, Khalil M, Jutley R. Uniportal video-assisted thoracoscopic surgery wedge lung biopsy in the diagnosis of interstitial lung diseases. J Thorac Cardiovasc Surg 2005;129:947–8.

6. Gonzalez D, Paradela M, Garcia J, et al. Single-port video-assisted thoracoscopic lobectomy. Interact Cardiovasc Thorac Surg 2011;12:514–5.

7. Gonzalez-Rivas D, Paradela M, Fernandez R, et al. Uniportal video-assisted thoracoscopic lobectomy: two years of experience. Ann Thorac Surg 2013; 95:426–32.

8. Sihoe ADL. The evolution of minimally invasive thoracic surgery: implications for the practice of uniportal thoracoscopic surgery. J Thorac Dis 2014; 6(Suppl 6):S604–17.

9. Gonzalez-Rivas D, Lopez D. Teaching thoracoscopic surgery around the world. 2014. Available at: https://www.youtube.com/watch?v=u-LjCWzvvuA. Accessed January 30, 2017.

10. Sihoe DLA. Opportunities and challenges for thoracic surgery collaborations in China: a commentary. J Thorac Dis 2016;8:S414–26.

11. Sihoe DLA. Reasons not to perform uniportal VATS lobectomy. J Thorac Dis 2016;8:S333–43.

12. Gonzalez-Rivas D, Delgado M, Fieira E, et al. Single-port video-assisted thoracoscopic lobectomy with pulmonary artery reconstruction. Interact Cardiovasc Thorac Surg 2013;17:889–91.

13. Gonzalez-Rivas D, Fieira E, Delgado M, et al. Is uniportal thoracoscopic surgery a feasible approach for advanced stages of non-small cell lung cancer? J Thorac Dis 2014;6:641–8.

14. Sihoe ADL. The evolution of VATS lobectomy. In: Cardoso P, editor. Topics in thoracic surgery. Rijeka (Croatia): Intech; 2011. p. 181–210.

15. Landreneau RJ, Mack MJ, Hazelrigg SR, et al. Prevalence of chronic pain after pulmonary resection by thoracotomy or video-assisted thoracic surgery. J Thorac Cardiovasc Surg 1994;107: 1079–86.

16. Kirby TJ, Mack MJ, Landreneau RJ, et al. Lobectomy video-assisted thoracic surgery versus

muscle-sparing thoracotomy: a randomized trial. J Thorac Cardiovasc Surg 1995;109:997–1002.

17. Nomori H, Horio H, Naruke T, et al. What is the advantage of a thoracoscopic lobectomy over a limited thoracotomy procedure for lung cancer surgery? Ann Thorac Surg 2001;72:879–84.

18. Yim APC, Landreneau RJ, Izzat MB, et al. Is video assisted thoracoscopic lobectomy a unified approach? Ann Thorac Surg 1998;66:1155–8.

19. Shigemura N, Akashi A, Nakagiri T, et al. Complete vs assisted thoracoscopic approach. A prospective randomized trial comparing a variety of video-assisted thoracoscopic lobectomy techniques. Surg Endosc 2004;18:1492–7.

20. Shigemura N, Akashi A, Funaki S, et al. Long-term outcomes after a variety of video-assisted thoracoscopic lobectomy approaches for clinical stage IA lung cancer: a multi-institutional study. J Thorac Cardiovasc Surg 2006;132:507–12.

21. Nagarajani R. Patient dies during live demo surgery at AIIMS, sparks ethics row. The Times of India. 2015. Available at: http://timesofindia.indiatimes.com/india/Patient-dies-during-live-demo-surgery-at-AIIMS-sparks-ethics-row/articleshow/48407921.cms. Accessed February 6, 2017.

22. Contraindication. Merriam-Webster.com. Merriam-Webster, n.d. Web. Available at: https://www.merriam-webster.com/dictionary/contraindication. Accessed February 6, 2017.

23. McElnay PJ, Molyneux M, Krishnadas R, et al. Pain and recovery are comparable after either uniportal and multiport video assisted thoracoscopic lobectomy: an observation study. Eur J Cardiothorac Surg 2015;47:912–5.

24. Chung JH, Choi YS, Cho JH, et al. Uniportal video-assisted thoracoscopic lobectomy: an alternative to conventional thoracoscopic lobectomy in lung cancer surgery? Interact Cardiovasc Thorac Surg 2015;20:813–9.

25. Wang BY, Liu CY, Hsu PK, et al. Single-incision versus multiple-incision thoracoscopic lobectomy and segmentectomy: a propensity-matched analysis. Ann Surg 2015;261:793–9.

26. Zhu Y, Liang M, Wu W, et al. Preliminary results of single-port versus triple-port complete thoracoscopic lobectomy for non-small cell lung cancer. Ann Transl Med 2015;3(7):92.

27. Liu CC, Shih CS, Pennarun N, et al. Transition from a multiport technique to a single-port technique for lung cancer surgery: is lymph node dissection inferior using the single-port technique? Eur J Cardiothorac Surg 2016;49:i64–72.

28. Hirai K, Takeuchi S, Usuda J. Single-incision thoracoscopic surgery and conventional video-assisted thoracoscopic surgery: a retrospective comparative study of perioperative clinical outcomes. Eur J Cardiothorac Surg 2016;49:i37–41.

29. Shen Y, Wang H, Feng M, et al. Single- versus multiple-port thoracoscopic lobectomy for lung cancer: a propensity-matched study. Eur J Cardiothorac Surg 2016;49:i48–53.

30. Mu JW, Gao SG, Xue Q, et al. A matched comparison study of uniportal versus triportal thoracoscopic lobectomy and sublobectomy for early-stage nonsmall cell lung cancer. Chin Med J 2015;128:2731–5.

31. Sihoe ADL, Yim APC. Video-assisted pulmonary resections. In: Patterson GA, Cooper JD, Deslauriers J, et al, editors. Thoracic surgery. 3rd Edition. Philadelphia: Elsevier; 2008. p. 970–88.

32. Park JS, Kim HK, Choi YS, et al. Unplanned conversion to thoracotomy during video-assisted thoracic surgery lobectomy does not compromise the surgical outcome. World J Surg 2011;35(3):590–5.

33. Yim AP, Liu HP, Hazelrigg SR, et al. Thoracoscopic operations on reoperated chests. Ann Thorac Surg 1998;65(2):328–30.

34. Gómez-Caro A, Roca Calvo MJ, Lanzas JT, et al. The approach of fused fissures with fissureless technique decreases the incidence of persistent air leak after lobectomy. Eur J Cardiothorac Surg 2007;31:203–8.

35. Sihoe AD, Chawla S, Paul S, et al. Technique for delivering large tumors in video-assisted thoracoscopic lobectomy. Asian Cardiovasc Thorac Ann 2014;22:319–28.

36. Nakanishi K. Video-assisted thoracic surgery lobectomy with bronchoplasty for lung cancer: initial experience and techniques. Ann Thorac Surg 2007;84:191–5.

37. Mahtabifard A, Fuller CB, McKenna RJ Jr. Video-assisted thoracic surgery sleeve lobectomy: a case series. Ann Thorac Surg 2008;85:S729–32.

38. Liu J, Cui F, He J. Non-intubated video-assisted thoracoscopic surgery anatomical resections: a new perspective for treatment of lung cancer. Ann Transl Med 2015;3(8):102.

39. Sihoe ADL. What is VATS? Asia Thoracoscopic Surgery Education Program. 2014. Available at: http://www.myatep.org/. Accessed January 30, 2017.

40. Sihoe DLA. Clinical pathway for videoassisted thoracic surgery: the Hong Kong story. J Thorac Dis 2016;8:S1222.

41. Sihoe ADL, Hiranandani R, Wong H, et al. Operating on a suspicious lung mass without a pre-operative tissue diagnosis: pros and cons. Eur J Cardiothorac Surg 2013;44:231–7.

42. Sihoe DLA. Uniportal videoassisted thoracic surgery (VATS) lobectomy. Ann Cardiothorac Surg 2016;5:133–44.

43. Gonzalez-Rivas D, Fernandez R, Fieira E, et al. Uniportal video-assisted thoracoscopic bronchial sleeve lobectomy: first report. J Thorac Cardiovasc Surg 2013;145:1676–7.

44. Rocco G, Romano V, Accardo R, et al. Awake single-access (uniportal) video-assisted thoracoscopic surgery for peripheral pulmonary nodules in a complete ambulatory setting. Ann Thorac Surg 2010;89:1625–7.

45. Gonzalez-Rivas D, Fernandez R, de la Torre M, et al. Uniportal video-assisted thoracoscopic left upper lobectomy under spontaneous ventilation. J Thorac Dis 2015;7(3):494–5.

46. Blackmon SH, Cooke DT, Whyte R, et al. The Society of Thoracic Surgeons Expert Consensus Statement: a tool kit to assist thoracic surgeons seeking privileging to use new technology and perform advanced procedures in general thoracic surgery. Ann Thorac Surg 2016;101(3):1230–7.

47. Mei J, Pu Q, Liao H, et al. A novel method for troubleshooting vascular injury during anatomic thoracoscopic pulmonary resection without conversion to thoracotomy. Surg Endosc 2013;27(2):530–7.

48. Kamiyoshihara M, Nagashima T, Igai H, et al. Unanticipated troubles in video-assisted thoracic surgery: a proposal for the classification of troubleshooting. Asian J Endosc Surg 2012;5(2):69–77.

49. Zhou W, Chen X, Zhang H, et al. Video-assisted thoracic surgery lobectomy for unexpected pathologic N2 non-small cell lung cancer. Thorac Cancer 2013;4:287–94.

50. Kim HK, Choi YS, Kim J, et al. Outcomes of unexpected pathologic N1 and N2 disease after video-assisted thoracic surgery lobectomy for clinical stage I non-small cell lung cancer. J Thorac Cardiovasc Surg 2010;140(6):1288–93.

51. Sihoe ADL, Luo Q, Shao G, et al. Uniportal thoracoscopic lobectomy for intralobar pulmonary sequestration. J Cardiothorac Surg 2016;11:27.

52. Samson P, Guitron J, Reed MF, et al. Predictors of conversion to thoracotomy for video-assisted thoracoscopic lobectomy: a retrospective analysis and the influence of computed tomography-based calcification assessment. J Thorac Cardiovasc Surg 2013;145(6):1512–8.

Subxiphoid Uniportal Video-Assisted Thoracoscopic Surgery Procedure

Takashi Suda, MD

KEYWORDS

• Subxiphoid • Thymectomy • Pulmonary • Lung • Surgery

KEY POINTS

- In recent years, the subxiphoid uniportal video-assisted thoracoscopic surgery approach has been used to avoid intercostal nerve damage in the field of thoracic surgery.
- A subxiphoid single-port thymectomy does not require sternotomy; it is associated with lesser pain because there is no intercostal nerve damage; and it provides aesthetically excellent outcomes.
- A subxiphoid single-port bilateral lung-wedge resection can be performed synchronously and, thus, does not cause intercostal nerve damage and excels in aesthetic outcomes.
- The subxiphoid single-port approach is a minimally invasive approach for thoracic surgery; specific technical development of the thoracoscopic instrumentation can yield improved operability resulting in wider acceptance of the technique.

 Video content accompanies this article at http://www.thoracic.theclinics.com.

INTRODUCTION

Minimally invasive surgery is currently adopted in many surgical fields because it imposes less physical stress on patients. Almost all procedures in the field of thoracic surgery, such as for lung cancer and mediastinal tumors, are undertaken through video-assisted thoracoscopic surgery (VATS).[1,2] In general, VATS is performed by inserting ports into small intercostal incisions made at 3 sites to 4 sites in the lateral aspect of the chest.[3,4] The lateral chest approach, however, via intercostal spaces, from the lateral to anterior chest region, corresponding to the intercostal space where a port was inserted, is associated with intercostal nerve damage that causes numbness and pain, which can persist for several months.[5] In recent

years, the subxiphoid approach has been used to avoid intercostal nerve damage. In 2012, the author and colleagues reported a single-port thymectomy by a subxiphoid approach.[6] Because this method does not require sternotomy, it is associated with lesser pain because there is no intercostal nerve damage and provides excellent cosmesis because only a single 3-cm abdominal skin incision is made. Furthermore, in 2014, the author and colleagues reported synchronous resection of bilateral pulmonary metastases by bilateral lung-wedge resection for bilateral metastatic lung tumors with a single 3-cm subxiphoid incision.[7] In this method, a bilateral lung-wedge resection is performed synchronously without an intercostal approach and, thus, does not cause

Conflict of Interest: None declared.
Division of Thoracic Surgery, Fujita Health University School of Medicine, 1-98 Dengakugakubo Kutsukake, Toyoake, Aichi 470-1192, Japan
E-mail address: suda@fujita-hu.ac.jp

Thorac Surg Clin 27 (2017) 381–386
http://dx.doi.org/10.1016/j.thorsurg.2017.06.006

intercostal nerve damage and provides excellent cosmesis, resulting in great advantage to patients. At present, this surgical technique is applied for resection of bilateral pulmonary metastases and in bullectomy for bilateral pneumothorax.

This report describes the author and colleagues' surgical technique for a single-port thymectomy and bilateral lung-wedge resection through the subxiphoid approach.

SURGICAL TECHNIQUES
Subxiphoid Uniportal Video-Assisted Thoracoscopic Surgery Thymectomy

Preoperative planning
This approach is adapted for thymomectomy and extended thymectomy for anterior mediastinal tumors or ablation of the thymic tissue for myasthenia gravis. In addition, tumors measuring up to 10 cm in size can be surgically removed provided that the initial skin incision is extended for tumor removal. This approach also enables a combined partial lung resection using a stapler. When the tumor invades the pericardium, or when suturing is required at any stage of the procedure, conversion to subxiphoid dual-port or subxiphoid triple-port thymectomy—with 1 to 2 additional ports in the precordial intercostal space—or subxiphoid robotic thymectomy[8] using the da Vinci Surgical System (Intuitive Surgical, Sunnyvale, California) becomes necessary.[9] In cases of suspected vascular infiltration, a median sternotomy is generally performed; however, if the brachiocephalic vein is partially transected by the stapler, a subxiphoid dual-port or subxiphoid robotic thymectomy can also be considered.

Preparation and patient positioning
Under general anesthesia, ventilation is usually provided through single-lumen endotracheal intubation. In general, 1-lung ventilation is unnecessary; however, when there is pulmonary invasion of the tumor necessitating partial lung resection, a double-lumen endotracheal tube is used. Artificial ventilation is performed using the pressure-controlled method. The patient is placed supine with the legs separated. Hypercapnia because of CO_2 insufflation is managed by increasing the respiratory rate. Positive end-expiratory pressure is not used to ensure the lungs do not become inflated. Epidural anesthesia is not used. In consideration of possible damage to, or clamping of, the brachiocephalic vein, the peripheral infusion route is secured by incannulating the right hand or foot.

Surgical procedure
A transverse or vertical 3-cm incision is made 1 cm below the xiphoid process. Transverse incisions follow the Langer lines of the skin to obviate a surgical scar (Video 1). Vertical incisions can easily be extended for tumor removal impeded by its size. Using an electric scalpel, the rectus abdominis is dissected at its attachment to the xiphoid process, and the lower portion of the thymus is detached from the posterior aspect of the sternum blindly through digital blunt dissection. There is no need to dissect the xiphoid process. An incision of approximately 5 mm is made caudally on the fascia of the rectus abdominis; then a space is created blindly using the finger to insert the GelPOINT Mini (Applied Medical, Rancho Santa Margarita, California)—a port for single-port surgery. This step requires caution to prevent peritoneal rupture, to avoid the entry of CO_2 into the abdominal cavity during surgery, with resultant abdominal distension and difficulty in surgical manipulations. The GelPOINT Mini with 3 small 10-mm ports is inserted into the incision (**Fig. 1**), and CO_2 insufflation at 8 mm Hg is performed. The surgeon stands between the legs of the patient during the surgery. The assistant stands to the right of the patient to operate the thoracoscope. The author and colleagues use a rigid thoracoscope 5 mm in diameter with a 30° oblique view. Initially, the thymus is detached from the posterior aspect of the sternum and up to the neck. Although not always possible, opening the mediastinal pleura is avoided. To verify the location of the phrenic nerve, both mediastinal pleural folds are incised and the thoracic cavity is exposed bilaterally. Holding a 36-cm SILS Clinch (Covidien, Mansfield, Massachusetts) forceps for single-port surgery in the left hand and a 37-cm LigaSure Maryland-type (Covidien) device in the right hand, the surgeon detaches the thymus from the pericardium (**Fig. 2**). When using

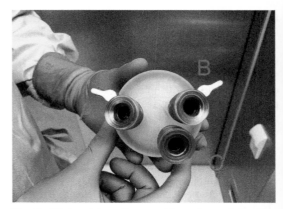

Fig. 1. Miniport insertion position. A, port for the camera scope; B, port for the surgeon's left hand; and C, port for the surgeon's right hand.

mediastinal pleura is dissected along and anterior to the right phrenic nerve. The proximal side of the left brachiocephalic vein and medial side of the right brachiocephalic vein of the neck are exposed. The thymus is detached from the pericardium caudal to the brachiocephalic veins. The bilateral superior poles of the thymus at the neck are detached from the brachiocephalic artery and the trachea. Caution should be exercised to not damage the inferior thyroid vein. By gently pulling to either side, the thymus is dissected with an energy device used to divide the thymic veins in the sequential order, thereby completing the thymectomy. The resected thymus is placed in a bag and extracted from the body through the subxiphoid incision. It is preferable to use a bag with no frame because the direction of the forceps used to extract a framed bag may become tangential to its mouth, making it difficult to place the resected thymus into the bag. A 20F drain is inserted into the mediastinum and it is usually removed on the following day. As a rule, patients is discharged home on the third postoperative day.

Subxiphoid Single-Port Bilateral Lung-Wedge Resection

Preoperative planning
Bilateral wedge resection is used in bilateral metastatic lung tumors and bilateral pneumothorax. Considering the advantage of excellent cosmetic outcome and absence of intercostal nerve damage, this technique may be adapted for unilateral lung-wedge resection. Because intraprocedural palpation is not possible, marking is necessary when resecting pulmonary nodules unless the mass is not directly beneath the pleura.

Preparation and patient positioning
Patients are placed supine with the legs separated. The operating table could tilt during surgery; therefore, the patient should be secured to the table to prevent a fall. The video monitor is placed at the head of the patient. The surgery is performed under general anesthesia with 1-lung ventilation. In case of hypoxemia or hypercapnia secondary to CO_2 insufflation and single-lung ventilation, the respiratory rate is increased and CO_2 insufflation is not performed. Epidural anesthesia is not administered.

Surgical procedure
As with the subxyphoid single-port thymectomy, a 3-cm skin incision is made 1 cm below the xiphoid process, the GelPOINT Mini is attached, and a 12-mm port is inserted into the main port that is used to insert the stapler (Video 2). After CO_2

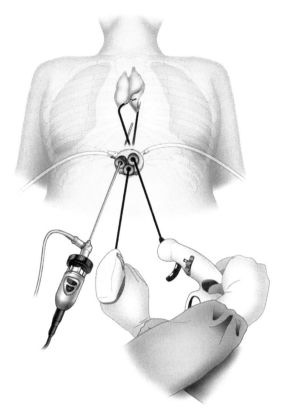

Fig. 2. Subxiphoid single-port thymectomy. The thymus is grasped using forceps for single-port surgery in the left hand, and the thymus is detached from the pericardium using the vessel-sealing device in the right hand.

LigaSure, to avoid damage to the pericardium and blood vessels, the electrocautery and cut function must be used only after the thymus has been dissected bluntly from the pericardium and blood vessels. When operating on the left lobe of the thymus, the tip of the SILS Clinch is bent toward the right, thereby pulling the thymus to the right hemithorax. Then, the surgeon changes hands, crossing them over, to detach the left lobe with LigaSure in the right hand. In contrast, for operations of the right lobe of the thymus, the tip of the SILS Clinch is bent to the left, thereby pulling the thymus to the left hemithorax. Then, the thymus is detached using LigaSure in the right hand; however, in this case, the surgeon does not need to cross hands over to extract the thymus.[10] The mediastinal pleura is dissected along and anterior to the left phrenic nerve up to the neck. The superficial fatty tissue near the left brachiocephalic vein is dissected from the surface of the thymus and the left brachiocephalic vein is carefully exposed. Similarly to the right side, the insufflation, the lower portion of the thymus is detached from the sternum using LigaSure. Although the author and colleagues use LigaSure, this procedure can be potentially performed using a normal electrical scalpel and forceps. The mediastinal pleura is dissected, and the thoracic cavity is exposed bilaterally. Similarly to the thymic procedure, for resection of the left lung, the tip of the SILS Clinch is bent toward the right, thereby pulling the lung upward and to the right; then the surgeon crosses hands over to perform lung-wedge resection using the stapler with a bent tip in the right hand (**Fig. 3**). In contrast, for operations of the right lung, the tip of SILS Clinch is bent to the left, thereby pulling the right lung to the left of the patient in an upward direction and lung-wedge resection is performed using the stapler held in the right hand, without a need to cross hands over. In uniportal surgery, if the forceps used to grasp the lung and stapler have a flexible, artculating tip, interference between instruments can be prevented. When the resection site is situated dorsally, tilting the surgical table so as to place the patient in a semisupine position facilitates surgery. To test for pulmonary air leakage after resection, distilled water is poured into one side only. Caution should be exercised because pouring water in both hemithoraces can cause ventilatory

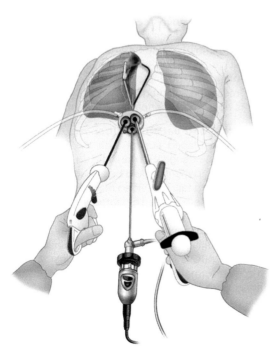

Fig. 3. Subxiphoid bilateral lung-wedge resection. The grasping forceps and stapler are used with a bent tip.

insufficiency. Two 20F drains are inserted through the wound below the xyphoid and directed one into each side of the thoracic cavity, and the wound is closed.

Clinical results in the literature

Most thoracic procedures can be undertaken through VATS.[1,2] From here on, VATS has 2 paths of development in the future. The first is to pursue more precise surgery while maintaining the current level of invasiveness (ie, robotic surgery), and the other is to pursue surgery with lesser invasiveness while maintaining the current level of surgical accuracy (ie, uniportal VATS surgery). In 2002, the use of uniportal VATS surgery was first reported in large numbers for sympathectomy[11]; then, in 2004 Rocco and colleagues[12] codified the uniportal VATS lung wedge resection. Furthermore, in 2011, Gonzalez-Rivas and colleagues[13] reported on uniportal VATS lobectomy as a procedure performed via a single incision in the lateral chest.[13] Thereafter, it was applied to more complex operations, such as bronchoplasty. Uniportal VATS, unlike conventional VATS, is performed via a single intercostal space and, therefore, is presumed to evoke less pain.[14,15]

In 2012, the author and colleagues reported a subxiphoid single-port thymectomy with CO_2 insufflation into the mediastinum and the use of single-port surgical instruments.[6] VATS for thymectomy is generally performed via the lateral chest approach via the intercostal space, which causes intercostal nerve damage in all patients, approximately 10% of whom experience lifelong persistent numbness and pain as the postthoracotomy pain syndrome.[5] Although VATS thymectomy via the lateral chest is associated with excellent cosmesis, it can cause pain and intercostal neuralgia, which may cast doubts on its lesser invasiveness compared with sternotomy. Advantages of the subxiphoid single-port approach include avoidance of sternal division and intercostal neuropathy as well as excellent cosmetic outcomes. Compared with VATS thymectomy via the lateral chest approach, the subxiphoid single-port approach has a shorter surgical duration, lesser estimated blood loss, shorter hospital stay, and less as well as shorter administration duration of postoperative analgesia.[16] Furthermore, compared with VATS thymectomy by a lateral chest approach, this method easily allows for a prompt verification of the location of bilateral phrenic nerves and secures a superior visualization of the upper poles of thymus. The disadvantage of subxiphoid single-port approach is the limited maneuverability. The author and colleagues believe this method offers considerable patient benefit and, thus, should be included in the thoracic surgical armamentarium. For surgeons adopting this surgical technique for the first time, it is recommended to insert a subxiphoid port initially and then add a 5-mm port into the left, right, or bilateral fifth intercostal space(s) after dissection of mediastinal pleura and opening of the thoracic cavity.[7] Doing so will greatly improve surgical maneuverability and safety.

In 2014, the author and colleagues reported on subxyphoid single-port bilateral resection of pulmonary metastases.[7] In the generally performed lateral approach for bilateral pulmonary nodules and bullae, in elderly or high-risk patients, the surgery is performed sequentially in 2 stages. In the first stage, ports are inserted at 3 sites on 1 side and, after performing lung-wedge resection, surgery is performed on the contralateral side. Postoperatively, 6 wounds remain on both sides of the chest, and intercostal nerve damage on both sides of the chest can cause numbness and pain. Conversely, with bilateral lung-wedge resection by single-port subxyphoid approach, there is only 1 incision and no intercostal nerve damage, and bilateral surgery can be performed in the same procedure. Therefore, the technique has the benefit of less invasiveness for patients. A problem with this procedure is that lung resection on the posterior side is difficult; however, by tilting the surgical table to place the patient in a semisupine position, and using grasping forceps and a stapler with a bendable tip, lung resection can be performed at almost all sites.

In 2014, Liu and colleagues[17] reported a single-port lobectomy and lymph node dissection by the subxyphoid approach for lung cancer. Factors impairing widespread acceptance of this least invasive lung cancer surgical technique could include the shortcomings of single-port surgery, associated with impaired maneuverability. Advanced modifications of these instruments, together with the emergence of recently developed robot-assisted surgical systems for single-port surgery, may compensate for these shortcomings and enable less-invasive surgery, including the subxyphoid approach. From these perspectives, it can easily be anticipated that single-port surgery by the subxyphoid approach may become even more important as a standardized approach for minimally invasive thoracic surgery in the future.

SUMMARY

Surgical techniques for single-port thymectomy and bilateral lung-wedge resection by the subxiphoid approach are reported. The subxiphoid single-port approach is a minimally invasive approach for thoracic surgery that can avoid intercostal nerve damage and, if supported by future technical development of instruments, can improve operability, resulting in wider acceptance of the technique.

SUPPLEMENTARY DATA

Supplementary data related to this article can be found at http://dx.doi.org/10.1016/j.thorsurg. 2017.06.006.

REFERENCES

1. McKenna RJ Jr, Houck W, Fuller CB. Video-assisted thoracic surgery lobectomy: experience with 1,100 cases. Ann Thorac Surg 2006;81(2):421–6.
2. Suda T, Kitamura Y, Hasegawa S, et al. Video-assisted thoracoscopic extrapleural pneumonectomy for malignant pleural mesothelioma. J Thorac Cardiovasc Surg 2007;134(4):1088–9.
3. Landreneau RJ, Dowling RD, Castillo WM, et al. Thoracoscopic resection of an anterior mediastinal tumor. Ann Thorac Surg 1992;54(1):142–4.
4. Sugarbaker DJ. Thoracoscopy in the management of anterior mediastinal masses. Ann Thorac Surg 1993;56:653–6.
5. Kehlet H, Jensen TS, Woolf CJ. Persistent postsurgical pain: risk factors and prevention. Lancet 2006;367(9522):1618–25.
6. Suda T, Sugimura H, Tochii D, et al. Single-port Thymectomy through an Infrasternal Approach. Ann Thorac Surg 2012;93(1):334–6.
7. Suda T, Ashikari S, Tochii S, et al. Single-incision subxiphoid approach for bilateral metastasectomy. Ann Thorac Surg 2014;97(2):718–9.
8. Suda T, Ashikari S, Tochii D, et al. Dual-port thymectomy using subxiphoid approach. Gen Thorac Cardiovasc Surg 2014;62(9):570–2.
9. Suda T, Tochii D, Tochii S, et al. Trans-subxiphoid robotic thymectomy. Interact Cardiovasc Thorac Surg 2015;20(5):669–71.
10. Suda T. Single-port thymectomy using a subxiphoid approach-surgical technique. Ann Cardiothorac Surg 2016;5(1):56–8.
11. Lardinois D, Ris HB. Minimally invasive video-endoscopic sympathectomy by use of a transaxillary single port approach. Eur J Cardiothorac Surg 2002;21(1):67–70.
12. Rocco G, Martin-Ucar A, Passera E. Uniportal VATS wedge pulmonary resections. Ann Thorac Surg 2004;77:726.
13. Gonzalez-Rivas D, de la Torre M, Fernandez R, et al. Single-port video-assisted thoracoscopic left upper lobectomy. Interact Cardiovasc Thorac Surg 2011; 13(5):539–41.

14. Gonzalez-Rivas D, Fernandez R, Fieira E, et al. Uni-portal video-assisted thoracoscopic bronchial sleeve lobectomy: first report. J Thorac Cardiovasc Surg 2013;145(6):1676–7.

15. Rocco G, Martucci N, La Manna C, et al. Ten-year experience on 644 patients undergoing single-port (uniportal) video-assisted thoracoscopic surgery. Ann Thorac Surg 2013;96(2):434–8.

16. Suda T, Hachimaru A, Tochii D, et al. Video assisted thoracoscopic thymectomy versus subxiphoid single-port thymectomy: initial results. Eur J Cardio-thorac Surg 2016;49:i54–8.

17. Liu CC, Wang BY, Shih CS, et al. Subxiphoid single-incision thoracoscopic left upper lobec-tomy. J Thorac Cardiovasc Surg 2014;148(6):3250–1.

Uniportal Video-Assisted Thoracoscopic Surgery Segmentectomy

Hyun Koo Kim, MD, PhD[a],*, Kook Nam Han, MD, PhD[b]

KEYWORDS

- Uniportal VATS • Single-port VATS • Non-small cell lung cancer • Sublobar resection
- Segmentectomy

KEY POINTS

- A uniportal approach to video-assisted thoracoscopic surgery (VATS) segmentectomy may be feasible, with minimal trauma owing to a minimal incision, regardless of the location of the lesion.
- Specific techniques for lesion localization and identification of intersegmental plane are essential to achieve the best operative results during VATS segmentectomy.
- Long-term outcomes using this alternative VATS technique for early stage lung cancer should be monitored.

INTRODUCTION

Since the introduction of lung segmentectomy for benign lesions in 1939, technical advances in thoracic surgery have changed the treatment of early stage non–small cell lung cancer (NSCLC).[1–3] The indications for segmentectomy include solitary pulmonary nodules,[4] infectious lung diseases with limited involvement,[5] and early stage lung malignancy.[6,7] Patients with poor cardiopulmonary reserve, insufficient for lobectomy, are also candidates for segmentectomy, to preserve normal lung parenchyma and reduce postoperative morbidity.[6] In addition, with the use of computed tomography (CT) for lung cancer screening, the detection of small tumors without nodal involvement is increasing. Moreover, lobectomy may be contraindicated in high-risk elderly patients.[8,9]

A randomized surgical trial for NSCLC (<3 cm), reported by the Lung Cancer Study Group in 1995, found an increased rate of locoregional recurrence with limited resection compared with lobectomy (8.6% vs 2.2%, respectively),[10] and concluded that lobectomy should be the standard for patients with stage IA lung cancer. However, recent trials have shown that anatomic sublobar resection (segmentectomy and wedge resection) can achieve outcomes equivalent to lobectomy in selected patients with stage IA NSCLC.[11–13]

Video-assisted thoracoscopic surgery (VATS) has become the standard approach for thoracic procedures,[14] and is usually performed through 3 or 4 access ports, with minimal incisions and no rib spreading. This approach is associated with not only less postoperative pain and low morbidity and mortality in the immediate postoperative period, but also shorter duration of hospitalization and lower medical costs. In addition, VATS segmentectomy has been shown to yield equivalent oncologic results compared with lobectomy using open or VATS technique.[15,16] More recently, there has been renewed interest in a uniportal approach, which was introduced by some pioneers.[17,18] Most

a Department of Thoracic and Cardiovascular Surgery, Korea University Guro Hospital, Korea University College of Medicine, 148, Gurodong-ro, Guro-gu, Seoul, 08308, Republic of Korea; b Department of Thoracic and Cardiovascular Surgery, Korea University College of Medicine, 148, Gurodong-ro, Guro-gu, Seoul, 08308, Republic of Korea
* Corresponding author.
E-mail address: kimhyunkoo@korea.ac.kr

Thorac Surg Clin 27 (2017) 387–398
http://dx.doi.org/10.1016/j.thorsurg.2017.06.007
1547-4127/17/© 2017 Elsevier Inc. All rights reserved.

thoracic.theclinics.com

thoracic procedures using conventional multiport VATS can be performed through a single, minimal incision (3–5 cm), with acceptable outcomes in treating lung malignancies.[19,20] It has been reported that uniportal VATS is safe and feasible, even for complex procedures, such as sleeve resection,[21,22] segmentectomy,[23–25] and vascular reconstruction.[26,27] Studies on the uniportal VATS approach are ongoing, with many surgeons using their own methods and instruments for various thoracic diseases.[28,29] The potential benefits are reduced intercostal pain and better cosmetic results; moreover, some patients make preferential requests for VATS. However, despite being the least invasive approach for early lung cancer, few studies have reported the outcomes of uniportal VATS segmentectomy, and the evidence is still unclear. As surgical experience increases, the supporting evidence will address the potential benefits of this innovative method for early stage lung cancer.

Improved techniques for localization of small lung lesions during VATS could help to prevent inappropriate division of the intersegmental plane.[30–32] In this section, we report our clinical experiences and introduce the technical details of uniportal VATS segmentectomy, including preoperative localization techniques. In addition, we performed a literature review of the obstacles and potential complications associated with this minimally invasive procedure.

PATIENT SELECTION

The usual indications for lung segmentectomy include a tumor less than 2 cm in diameter without thoracic lymph node involvement, a small (<1 cm) ground glass opacity (<50%), or a benign lung disease with poor or even with normal pulmonary reserve, in which the goal is to preserve normal lung parenchyma.[12,33,34] There are no absolute exclusion criteria for uniportal VATS, although conventional multiport VATS might be more appropriate in selected patients with extensive adhesions. Theoretically, limited pulmonary wedge resection and segmentectomy seem to be well-matched to a limited incision approach such as uniportal VATS. Furthermore, the use of uniportal VATS with a small incision (2–3 cm) may be justified, because the resected specimen can be removed through the incision. Our indications for pulmonary segmentectomy include a solitary peripheral pulmonary nodule measuring 2 cm or less in the targeted segment, suspected cT1N0M0 lung cancer, and small (<1 cm) ground-glass opacities on chest CT (**Fig. 1**). Other indications include a metastatic or benign pulmonary tumor that cannot be accessed by wedge

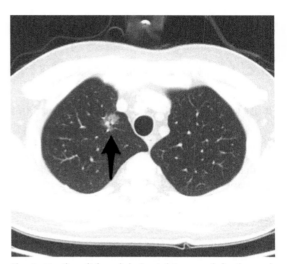

Fig. 1. Partly solid nodule in right upper lobe (*arrow*). Clinical T1aN0 non–small cell lung cancer.

resection, or inflammatory disease that is resectable through segmentectomy instead of lobectomy, thereby preserving lung parenchyma in patients with poor pulmonary reserve.

TECHNIQUE
Preoperative Localization

Chest CT with 3-dimensional reconstruction can be helpful in planning surgery. The possibility of a fused fissure and the anatomy of the segmental branches of the pulmonary artery and vein should be evaluated for a safe operation. In addition, preoperative localization with a radiotracer, coil, radioopaque marker, or a hook-wire may be indicated for small, nonpalpable nodules that are difficult to localize using a minimally invasive approach.[35–37] We routinely perform preoperative CT-guided localization of pulmonary tumors with the dual use of a hook-wire and lipiodol or a radioisotope to identify the intersegmental plane for a sufficient resection margin (>2 cm from the lesion) in candidates for pulmonary segmentectomy (**Fig. 2**).

However, if a pneumothorax or hemothorax had been caused by a previous percutaneous needle lung biopsy, or if there is sufficient resection distance from the intersegmental plane on CT, we do not perform localization. The advantage of dual localization is a higher lesion detection rate, even when a hook-wire is dislodged.[30] The localization technique is also used to identify the proper resection margin in deeper lesions. These procedures were performed 1 to 2 hours before surgery, and were guided by CT fluoroscopy. Intraoperative C-arm fluoroscopy was used to detect the lipiodol, and a gamma probe was used to detect radiotracer marking before segmental division (**Fig. 3**).

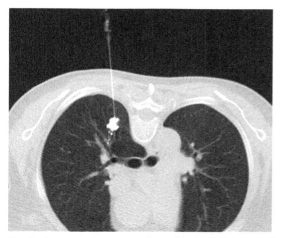

Fig. 2. Computed tomography-guided localization of lung nodule using lipiodol.

Localization techniques are evolving with technical advances. Electromagnetic navigational bronchoscopy is a good option for noninvasive localization,[38,39] because percutaneous injection can cause a hemothorax, pneumothorax,[40] or fatal embolism.[41] Such localized lung lesions can be detected using intraoperative C-arm fluoroscopy. A near-infrared fluorescent video surgical system might be a feasible option for localization of a lung lesion by direct view without C-arm fluoroscopy (**Fig. 4**).[42]

Positioning and Instrumentation

The basic anesthesia protocol and surgical techniques are similar to those used in previously

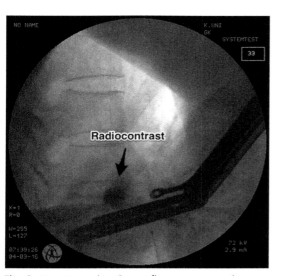

Fig. 3. Intraoperative C-arm fluoroscopy to detect a radiopaque marker (*arrow*).

reported uniportal VATS lobectomy.[43,44] The lateral decubitus position is standard. We make a 2- to 4-cm incision on the fifth intercostal space along the midaxillary line (**Fig. 5**). The position of the surgeon and the level of incision, however, might change, depending on the tumor location. To achieve better instrument performance, and to prevent wound contamination from the cancer, we always apply a wound protector at the port site (**Fig. 6**). In our experience, the surgeon was always positioned on the right side and the assistant on the left side of the patient (**Fig. 7**).

There are various approaches and positions for uniportal VATS, depending on the surgeon's preference. Gonzalez-Rivas et al reported that a wound retractor might limit the use of instrumentation during the procedure, and always stood anterior to the patient, with a port incision closer to the anterior axillary line. They emphasized that camera instrumentation is crucial for better operative performance and recommended that the camera should be fixed to the posterior edge of the port.[18,23] Wang and colleagues[45] performed uniportal VATS segmentectomy with a 3- to 5-cm incision on the fifth or sixth intercostal space in the anterior axillary line. They always stood anterior to the patient and routinely used a wound protector.

A 3.3- or 5-mm conventional thoracoscope, or a 10-mm thoracoscope with a 3-dimensional view, are used in our procedures (**Fig. 8**). A 3- or 5-mm curved, articulating endoscopic instruments, a 3- or 5-mm tailored grasper with the length of the shaft shortened, and a flexible and/or curved tip endostapler is used during the operations. To divide the pulmonary segmental vessel, we use a vascular 30-mm endostapler. In cases where it is impossible to insert the endostapler owing to a difficult angle, we use interlocking vascular clips (**Fig. 9**).

Identification of the Intersegmental Plane

It is important to achieve appropriate resection margins when the target disease is a malignant lesion. During open thoracotomy, surgeons usually palpate the lung nodule and adherent vascular structures to identify the complex lung segmental anatomy. However, in VATS, it is impossible to palpate the lung and demarcate the proper resection margin without tactile feedback.

Several groups have described the various techniques for the identification of the intersegmental plane during VATS segmentectomy. The inflation and deflation method is usually performed during segmentectomy. Tsubota[46] reported the inflation

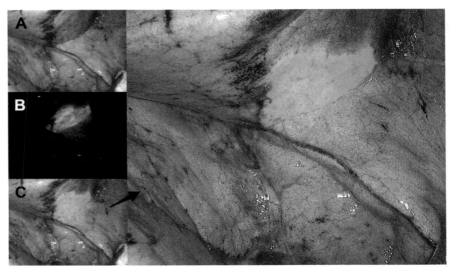

Fig. 4. Near-infrared fluorescence localization using indocyanine green (ICG). (*A*) Normal thoracoscopic image. (*B*) Near infrared fluorescence image. (*C*) Fusion image. *Arrow* indicates the enlarged picture from fusion image.

technique to identify the affected segments. Okada and colleagues[34] used a jet ventilation technique by selectively inflating the segmental bronchus to visualize the intersegmental plane. However, this technique requires a fiberoptic bronchoscope and a specialist for handling this device to the segmental and subsegmental bronchus during surgery.

Oizumi and colleagues[47,48] described the technique of 3-dimensional lung segmental color mapping from multislice CT angiography to understand the individual lung segmental anatomy and variations of the segmental vessels and bronchi. They reported a 98% completion rate for

segmentectomy using 3-dimensional reconstruction images. Also, they emphasized that the intersegmental vein could be a guide for the parenchymal dissection.

The recent development of near-infrared fluorescence technique using intraoperative injection of indocyanine green to the segmental pulmonary artery or directly to the segmental bronchus has been reported as a promising method in terms of visualization of the real-time segmental anatomy.[42,49,50] However, this technique requires a special fluorescence imaging system currently not in general use and needs direct injection of indocyanine green to the segmental artery

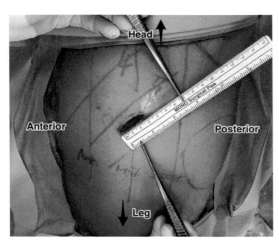

Fig. 5. Incision over the fifth intercostal space in the midaxillary line.

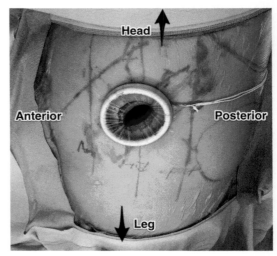

Fig. 6. Wound protector applied at port site to widen the port and prevent contamination from the specimen.

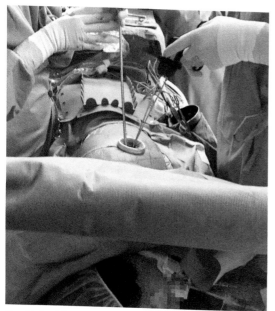

Fig. 7. Position and instrumentation during uniportal video-assisted thoracoscopic surgery.

or segmental bronchus intraoperatively by another doctor who can maneuver the fiberoptic bronchoscope.

TECHNIQUES FOR SEGMENTECTOMY
Right and Left Upper Lobe Apical and Posterior Segments

There are 3 lung segments in the right upper lobe: the apical, posterior, and anterior. Preoperative planning and understanding of segmental anatomy by the thoracic surgeon are essential first steps in uniportal VATS segmentectomy.

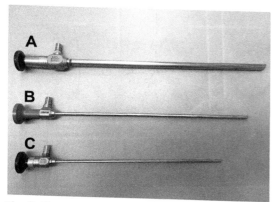

Fig. 8. Thoracoscopes used for uniportal surgery: (*A*) 10-mm 30°-angled thoracoscope, (*B*) 5-mm 30°-angled thoracoscope, and (*C*) 3.3-mm thoracoscope.

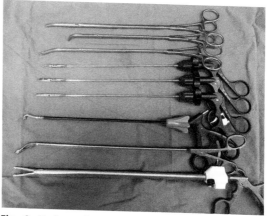

Fig. 9. Endoscopic instruments for uniportal video-assisted thoracoscopic surgery segmentectomy.

Preoperative CT is helpful for evaluation of common variants of segmental structures.[51] A 2- to 3-cm port can usually be created in the fourth or fifth intercostal space in the midaxillary or anterior axillary line to approach the upper lobe segmental structures.

The surgical view in uniportal VATS (direct view is similar to that of open thoracotomy) is different from that in conventional VATS (lateral view of the lung; **Fig. 10**).[52] Mobilization of the right upper lobe posteriorly can expose the upper lobar pulmonary veins (usually 3 divisions: superior, central, and middle lobar). The superior vein drains the posterior segment and lies deep to the posterior portion of the central segmental veins. Care must be taken in dividing the apical and posterior segmental veins because anatomic variants of the segmental artery and vein are usually present (**Fig. 11**).

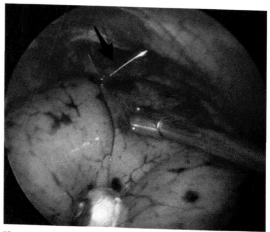

Fig. 10. Hook-wire (*arrow*) localization of apical lung lesion in right upper lobe.

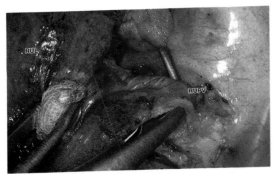

Fig. 11. Segmental branch of right upper pulmonary vein. RUL, right upper lobe; RUPV, right upper pulmonary vein.

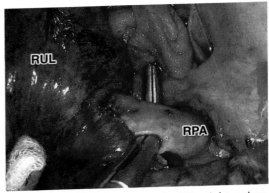

Fig. 13. Truncus anterior branch. RPA, right pulmonary artery; RUL, right upper lobe.

Dissection of the major fissure exposes the upper lobe pulmonary segmental arterial branch. The apical pulmonary segmental artery can then be exposed by dissection of the truncus anterior, which consists of the apical and anterior segmental arteries (Fig. 12). Mobilization of the upper lobe is helpful in exposing the truncus anterior branch near the azygos vein (Fig. 13). After transection of the apical and posterior segmental arteries, the upper lobar bronchus can be identified easily in a deeper location.

Lymph node excision around the upper lobar bronchus can facilitate the isolation of the 3 segmental bronchi (apical, posterior, and anterior). If there is no lymph node metastasis on frozen examination of the segmental lymph nodes, bronchial division is completed after identification of the correct bronchus (Fig. 14) by demarcating the intersegmental plane. Selective inflation with a pediatric fiberoptic bronchoscope is used to identify the intersegmental plane, after clamping the presumed apical or apicoposterior segmental bronchus (Fig. 15).

The intersegmental plane is usually identified by lung inflation after division of the segmental bronchus (Fig. 16). It is important to divide the intersegmental plane from the lung lesion with a proper resection margin. To achieve a proper resection margin for a subpleural lesion, stapling may be guided with finger palpation or a direct view.

In contrast, deeper lesions may require the use of localization technique to identify the proper resection margin. A hook-wire, fiducial, or radiopaque material should be injected or placed under preoperative CT guidance. Electromagnetic navigational bronchoscopy is a good option for noninvasive localization,[40] because percutaneous injection can cause a hemothorax or pneumothorax. In addition, because localized lung lesions can only be detected by intraoperative C-arm fluoroscopy, a near-infrared fluorescence video surgical system[44] might be a future application for visualization of the target lung lesion and the intersegmental plane by direct view without C-arm fluoroscopy (Fig. 17).

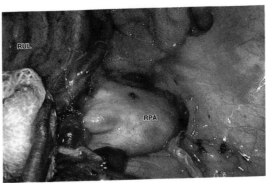

Fig. 12. Upper divisional branches of right pulmonary artery. RPA, right pulmonary artery; RUL, right upper lobe.

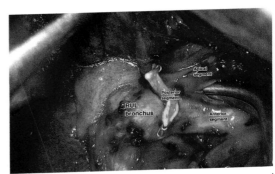

Fig. 14. Apical segmental bronchus and transected posterior segmental bronchus. RUL, right upper lobe.

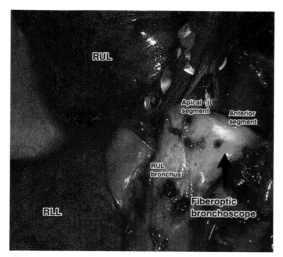

Fig. 15. Apical segmental bronchus (clamped) and fiber optic bronchoscope in anterior segmental bronchus (*arrow*). RLL, right lower lobe; RUL, right upper lobe.

Right and Left Lower Lobe Superior Segments

The position and port for the uniportal approach to these segments are the same as those for upper lobar segmentectomy. We prefer a 2- to 4-cm single incision in the midaxillary line, which is different from that used by other surgeons. The interlobar pulmonary artery can be identified from the entry of the single port. A complete fissure is usually dissected using electrocautery or endoscopic dissecting devices. An energy device is useful to divide an incomplete fissure, or a stapler can be used for fissure division. One can achieve full mobilization of the lower lobe by division of the inferior pulmonary ligament. After dissection of perivascular lymph nodes at the segmental vessel,

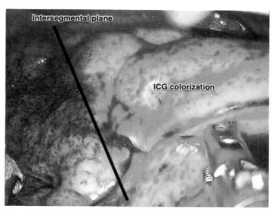

Fig. 17. Identification of intersegmental plane using near-infrared fluorescence system with intravenous injection of indocyanine green (ICG).

the superior segmental artery is divided with a vascular stapler or vascular clips. Care must be taken to identify the posterior ascending branch, because it may branch off the superior segmental artery before the transection. After division of the superior segmental artery, the superior segmental bronchus can be seen posteriorly (**Fig. 18**). Complete division of the major fissure helps to identify the superior segmental bronchus. In the uniportal surgical view, anterior traction on the lower lobe can expose the ventral column, and the superior segmental bronchus can be exposed by dissecting between the upper lobar bronchus and the bronchus intermedius (**Fig. 19**). In this position, subcarinal lymph nodes can also be dissected by traction on the lower lobe anteriorly. After full mobilization of the segmental bronchus, one can complete the division of the superior segmental bronchus with the lung inflation technique. The superior segmental vein can be identified by traction on the lower lobe anteriorly or superiorly, and

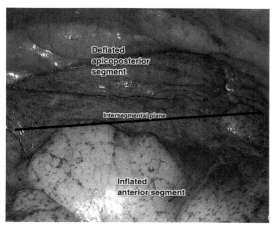

Fig. 16. Intersegmental plane between the apicoposterior and anterior segments.

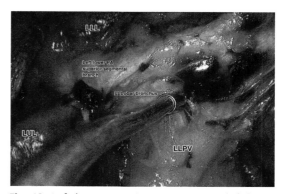

Fig. 18. Left lower superior segment. LLL, left lower lobe; LLPV, left lower pulmonary vein; LUL, left upper lobe; PA, pulmonary artery.

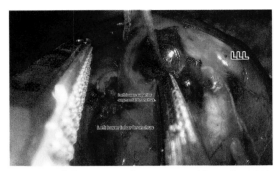

Fig. 19. Left lower superior segmental bronchus. LLL, left lower lobe.

divided with a vascular stapler or clips. The intersegmental plane is divided with the lung inflation technique.

Right and Left Lower Lobe Basal Segments

The position and port for the uniportal approach to the basal segments are the same as those for lower lobe superior segmentectomy. The basilar segmental artery is exposed by dissection of the fissure. Complete division of the major and minor fissures is helpful for dissection of the basilar artery and segmental bronchus. After transection of the basilar segmental artery, the basilar segmental bronchus can easily be dissected and divided. After stapling the basilar segmental bronchus with proper identification of the correct segment, basilar segmental veins can be exposed by traction on the lower lobe superiorly and posteriorly. The sequence of division for the bronchus and vein is not consistent, but is based on the surgeon's experience with the uniportal VATS technique. The basilar segmental vein is transected with vascular staplers or clips, with preservation of the superior segmental veins.

Left Upper Divisional Segment (Trisegment)

A 2- to 3-cm incision is created on the fifth intercostal space along the anterior axillary line (**Fig. 20**). The surgeon stands on the right side of the patient. The interlobar fissure is dissected and divided by electrocautery, energy device, or staplers to expose the posterior and lingular segmental pulmonary arteries. The common upper trunk can be identified by dissection of the mediastinal pleura after left upper lobe traction posteriorly. Interlobar and segmental lymph nodes should be excised by careful manipulation. The upper divisional pulmonary arteries can be exposed after the upper divisional veins are divided (**Fig. 21**), because there might be difficulty in passing the vascular stapler between the upper divisional

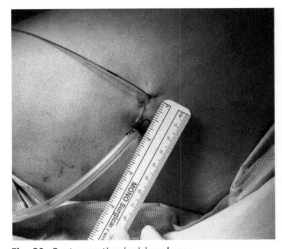

Fig. 20. Postoperative incisional scar.

vein and artery. Penrose-guided stapler insertion is helpful to avoid excessive tension on vascular structures during stapling. The upper divisional bronchus is exposed after the upper divisional artery and vein are divided. To divide the upper divisional segmental plane, fiberoptic bronchoscopy and selective jet inflation and deflation of the segmental bronchus can be used to demarcate the intersegmental plane between the upper division and the lingular segment.

Left Lingular Segment

The incision and preparation are the same as in the approach to upper divisional segmentectomy. The interlobar fissure is opened or dissected to expose the lingular branch artery, which usually originates from the interlobar artery. The lingular segmental vein can be isolated by dissection of the upper pulmonary vein by traction on the upper lobe posteriorly. It is advantageous to divide the lingular vein

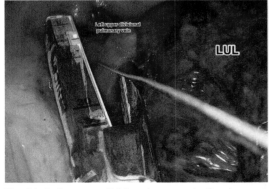

Fig. 21. Left upper divisional segment of pulmonary vein. LUL, left upper lobe.

first to expose the lingular segmental bronchus. The lingular segmental artery is divided using vascular staplers. Aberrant small vascular branches can be transected by vascular clips or energy devices.

RESULTS OF UNIPORTAL VIDEO-ASSISTED THORACOSCOPIC SURGERY SEGMENTECTOMY

The earliest report of uniportal VATS segmentectomy was published in 2012.[23] However, this approach has raised questions of adequacy regarding safety and oncologic outcomes.[45,53] There are no randomized trials or well-designed case-control studies of this approach, and only a few reports showing low-grade evidence.[23,24,45,54]

A few case reports and series have described ongoing surgical experiences, with only short-term follow-up and fewer than 50 cases in each report (**Table 1**). Gonzalez-Rivas and colleagues[55] have been publishing their experiences with uniportal VATS segmentectomy for NSCLC since 2012. They published the first case report of uniportal VATS segmentectomy as a combined procedure in a patient with a 1-cm nodule in the superior segment of the right lower lobe. They made a 3-cm incision in the fifth intercostal space in the anterior axillary line and did not use rib spreading. Their technique does not use a wound

protector and the surgeon always stands anterior to the patient. They performed 28 cases with a 2-day duration of stay (range, 1–6 days) and suggested that a uniportal VATS approach to segmentectomy might be a safe and feasible procedure with outcomes of morbidity and mortality equivalent to those of thoracotomy.

Wang and colleagues[54] published their experience with 27 procedures (11 uniportal and 16 multiport segmentectomies). They made a 3- to 5-cm incision on the sixth intercostal space along the anterior axillary line and routinely used a wound protector. Both the operator and the scope assistant stand anterior to the patient during the procedure. In propensity-matched analysis, they reported that the advantages of uniportal VATS segmentectomy compared with multiport VATS were shorter operative times, retrieval of more lymph nodes, and less intraoperative blood loss.

Han and colleagues[24,56] published a series of 30 patients with NSCLC or benign lesions in whom they attempted uniportal VATS segmentectomy. A 2- to 4-cm incision was used and there was no conversion to open thoracotomy. On follow-up, they reported that uniportal VATS segmentectomy showed lower morbidity and shorter duration of hospital stay compared with multiport VATS segmentectomy.

As noted, there are only a few case series of uniportal VATS segmentectomy, resulting in

Table 1
Literature published to date on uniportal VATS segmentectomy

Study, Year	No. of Patients	Study	Segment	Comments
Gonzalez-Rivas et al,[19,23] 2012	1	Case	Superior segment of RLL	Direct vision to target tissue Potentially less intercostal pain
Wang et al,[45] 2013	5	Case series	Basilar segment of LLL (1), lingular segment of LUL (4)	2 developed atelectasis Longer LOS than that of lobectomy
Gonzalez et al,[55] 2013	28	Case series	Not described	Shorter LOS Equivalent morbidity and mortality to that of thoracotomy
Wang et al,[54] 2015	11 (uniportal) vs 16 (multiport)	Propensity-matched analysis	Not described	Short operative time, more lymph nodes dissected, and less blood loss
Han et al,[24,56] 2016	30	Case series	All types of segments	Feasible
Han et al,[24,56] 2016	34 (uniportal) vs 11 (multiport)	Case control	All types of segments	Low morbidity and hospital stay
Lin et al,[57] 2016	32	Case series	Not described	Faster recovery

Abbreviations: LLL, left lower lobe; LOS, length of stay; LUL, left upper lobe; RLL, right lower lobe.

low-grade evidence. Currently, there seems to be no strong evidence supporting the superiority or inferiority of a uniportal VATS approach. Therefore, we can state that uniportal VATS segmentectomy for NSCLC or benign disease in selected patients is a safe and feasible procedure; however, oncologic outcomes should be compared with those for open thoracotomy or a multiport VATS approach, which seem to be equivalent. There is a need for future studies regarding this issue.

Moreover, the potential benefit for postoperative pain remains controversial. In contrast with the reports by proponents of uniportal VATS, Perna and colleagues[58] found no difference in early postoperative pain according to the number of ports during VATS. This issue should also be addressed in a well-designed randomized trial for comparison with multiport VATS. However, there may be some advantages in performing uniportal VATS if patients are better able to tolerate adjuvant chemotherapy after this procedure.

SUMMARY

Uniportal VATS segmentectomy is a technically demanding, but safe and feasible procedure for selected patients with both malignant and benign lesions. With proper selection of patients and the use of appropriate techniques and instruments, the surgeon can achieve better results, even with a uniportal approach. Although care must be taken during the learning phase, this least invasive approach seems to be an acceptable alternative to conventional VATS and open thoracotomy.

ACKNOWLEDGMENTS

This work was supported by a grant from the Korean Health Technology R&D Project, Ministry of Health & Welfare, Republic of Korea (A121074) and the National Research Foundation of Korea (NRF) grant funded by the Ministry of Education, Science and Technology (2015R1A2A2A04005760[A1]).

REFERENCES

1. Yan TD, Black D, Bannon PG, et al. Systematic review and meta-analysis of randomized and non-randomized trials on safety and efficacy of video-assisted thoracic surgery lobectomy for early-stage non-small-cell lung cancer. J Clin Oncol 2009; 27(15):2553–62.

2. Okada M, Koike T, Higashiyama M, et al. Radical sublobar resection for small-sized non-small cell lung cancer: a multicenter study. J Thorac Cardiovasc Surg 2006;132(4):769–75.

3. Okada M. Radical sublobar resection for small-diameter lung cancers. Thorac Surg Clin 2013; 23(3):301–11.

4. Schuchert MJ, Abbas G, Awais O, et al. Anatomic segmentectomy for the solitary pulmonary nodule and early-stage lung cancer. Ann Thorac Surg 2012;93(6):1780–5 [discussion: 6–7].

5. Mitchell JD, Yu JA, Bishop A, et al. Thoracoscopic lobectomy and segmentectomy for infectious lung disease. Ann Thorac Surg 2012;93(4):1033–9 [discussion: 9–40].

6. Jones DR, Stiles BM, Denlinger CE, et al. Pulmonary segmentectomy: results and complications. Ann Thorac Surg 2003;76(2):343–8 [discussion: 8–9].

7. Tsutani Y, Miyata Y, Nakayama H, et al. Oncologic outcomes of segmentectomy compared with lobectomy for clinical stage IA lung adenocarcinoma: propensity score-matched analysis in a multicenter study. J Thorac Cardiovasc Surg 2013;146(2): 358–64.

8. Pedersen JH, Ashraf H, Dirksen A, et al. The Danish randomized lung cancer CT screening trial–overall design and results of the prevalence round. J Thorac Oncol 2009;4(5):608–14.

9. National Lung Screening Trial Research Team, Aberle DR, Adams AM, Berg CD, et al. Reduced lung-cancer mortality with low-dose computed tomographic screening. N Engl J Med 2011; 365(5):395–409.

10. Ginsberg RJ, Rubinstein LV. Randomized trial of lobectomy versus limited resection for T1 N0 non-small cell lung cancer. Lung Cancer Study Group. Ann Thorac Surg 1995;60(3):615–22 [discussion: 22–3].

11. Martin-Ucar AE, Nakas A, Pilling JE, et al. A case-matched study of anatomical segmentectomy versus lobectomy for stage I lung cancer in high-risk patients. Eur J Cardiothorac Surg 2005;27(4): 675–9.

12. Koike T, Yamato Y, Yoshiya K, et al. Intentional limited pulmonary resection for peripheral T1 N0 M0 small-sized lung cancer. J Thorac Cardiovasc Surg 2003;125(4):924–8.

13. Smith CB, Swanson SJ, Mhango G, et al. Survival after segmentectomy and wedge resection in stage I non-small-cell lung cancer. J Thorac Oncol 2013; 8(1):73–8.

14. Yim AP. VATS major pulmonary resection revisited–controversies, techniques, and results. Ann Thorac Surg 2002;74(2):615–23.

15. Yang CF, D'Amico TA. Thoracoscopic segmentectomy for lung cancer. Ann Thorac Surg 2012;94(2): 668–81.

16. Shiraishi T, Shirakusa T, Iwasaki A, et al. Video-assisted thoracoscopic surgery (VATS) segmentectomy for small peripheral lung cancer tumors: intermediate results. Surg Endosc 2004;18(11):1657–62.

17. Rocco G, Martin-Ucar A, Passera E. Uniportal VATS wedge pulmonary resections. Ann Thorac Surg 2004;77(2):726–8.

18. Gonzalez-Rivas D, Paradela M, Fernandez R, et al. Uniportal video-assisted thoracoscopic lobectomy: two years of experience. Ann Thorac Surg 2013; 95(2):426–32.

19. Gonzalez-Rivas D, Paradela M, Fieira E, et al. Single-incision video-assisted thoracoscopic lobectomy: initial results. J Thorac Cardiovasc Surg 2012; 143(3):745–7.

20. Rocco G. One-port (uniportal) video-assisted thoracic surgical resections–a clear advance. J Thorac Cardiovasc Surg 2012;144(3):S27–31.

21. Andrade H, Joubert P, Vieira A, et al. Single-port right upper lobe sleeve lobectomy for a typical carcinoid tumour. Interact Cardiovasc Thorac Surg 2017; 24(2):315–6.

22. Gonzalez-Rivas D, Fernandez R, Fieira E, et al. Uniportal video-assisted thoracoscopic bronchial sleeve lobectomy: first report. J Thorac Cardiovasc Surg 2013;145(6):1676–7.

23. Gonzalez-Rivas D, Fieira E, Mendez L, et al. Single-port video-assisted thoracoscopic anatomic segmentectomy and right upper lobectomy. Eur J Cardiothorac Surg 2012;42(6):e169–71.

24. Han KN, Kim HK, Lee HJ, et al. Single-port video-assisted thoracoscopic pulmonary segmentectomy: a report on 30 cases. Eur J Cardiothorac Surg 2016; 49(Suppl 1):i42–7.

25. Shih CS, Liu CC, Liu ZY, et al. Comparing the postoperative outcomes of video-assisted thoracoscopic surgery (VATS) segmentectomy using a multi-port technique versus a single-port technique for primary lung cancer. J Thorac Dis 2016;8(Suppl 3):S287–94.

26. Gonzalez-Rivas D, Yang Y, Stupnik T, et al. Uniportal video-assisted thoracoscopic bronchovascular, tracheal and carinal sleeve resections. Eur J Cardiothorac Surg 2016;49(Suppl 1):i6–16.

27. Gonzalez-Rivas D, Delgado M, Fieira E, et al. Single-port video-assisted thoracoscopic lobectomy with pulmonary artery reconstruction. Interact Cardiovasc Thorac Surg 2013;17(5):889–91.

28. Hernandez-Arenas LA, Lin L, Yang Y, et al. Initial experience in uniportal subxiphoid video-assisted thoracoscopic surgery for major lung resections. Eur J Cardiothorac Surg 2016;50(6):1060–6.

29. Wu L, Lin L, Liu M, et al. Subxiphoid uniportal thoracoscopic extended thymectomy. J Thorac Dis 2015; 7(9):1658–60.

30. Park CH, Han K, Hur J, et al. Comparative effectiveness and safety of pre-operative lung localization for pulmonary nodules: a systematic review and meta-analysis. Chest 2016;151(2):316–28.

31. Finley RJ, Mayo JR, Grant K, et al. Preoperative computed tomography-guided microcoil localization of small peripheral pulmonary nodules: a prospective randomized controlled trial. J Thorac Cardiovasc Surg 2015;149(1):26–31.

32. Powell TI, Jangra D, Clifton JC, et al. Peripheral lung nodules: fluoroscopically guided video-assisted thoracoscopic resection after computed tomography-guided localization using platinum microcoils. Ann Surg 2004;240(3):481–8 [discussion: 8–9].

33. Okada M, Yoshikawa K, Hatta T, et al. Is segmentectomy with lymph node assessment an alternative to lobectomy for non-small cell lung cancer of 2 cm or smaller? Ann Thorac Surg 2001;71(3):956–60 [discussion: 61].

34. Okada M, Mimura T, Ikegaki J, et al. A novel video-assisted anatomic segmentectomy technique: selective segmental inflation via bronchofiberoptic jet followed by cautery cutting. J Thorac Cardiovasc Surg 2007;133(3):753–8.

35. Bellomi M, Veronesi G, Trifiro G, et al. Computed tomography-guided preoperative radiotracer localization of nonpalpable lung nodules. Ann Thorac Surg 2010;90(6):1759–64.

36. Galetta D, Bellomi M, Grana C, et al. Radio-guided localization and resection of small or ill-defined pulmonary lesions. Ann Thorac Surg 2015;100(4): 1175–80.

37. Chen S, Zhou J, Zhang J, et al. Video-assisted thoracoscopic solitary pulmonary nodule resection after CT-guided hookwire localization: 43 cases report and literature review. Surg Endosc 2011;25(6): 1723–9.

38. McWilliams A, Shaipanich T, Lam S. Fluorescence and navigational bronchoscopy. Thorac Surg Clin 2013;23(2):153–61.

39. Kalanjeri S, Gildea TR. Electromagnetic navigational bronchoscopy for peripheral pulmonary nodules. Thorac Surg Clin 2016;26(2):203–13.

40. Pittet O, Christodoulou M, Pezzetta E, et al. Video-assisted thoracoscopic resection of a small pulmonary nodule after computed tomography-guided localization with a hook-wire system. Experience in 45 consecutive patients. World J Surg 2007;31(3): 575–8.

41. Horan TA, Pinheiro PM, Araujo LM, et al. Massive gas embolism during pulmonary nodule hook wire localization. Ann Thorac Surg 2002;73(5):1647–9.

42. Han KN, Kim HK, Choi YH. Fluorescent thoracoscopic right upper apicoposterior segmentectomy for early lung cancer: real-time visualization of lymphatic flow and segmental anatomy using indocyanine green. STS 53rd Annual Meeting. George R. Brown Convention Center in Houston, Texas. January 21-25, 2017; Surgical Motion Picture Martinee; General Thoracic: Session.

43. Kim HK, Sung HK, Lee HJ, et al. The feasibility of a Two-incision video-assisted thoracoscopic lobectomy. J Cardiothorac Surg 2013;8:88.

44. Kim HK, Choi YH. The feasibility of single-incision video-assisted thoracoscopic major pulmonary resection performed by surgeons experienced with a two-incision technique. Interact Cardiovasc Thorac Surg 2015;20(3):310–5.

45. Wang BY, Tu CC, Liu CY, et al. Single-incision thoracoscopic lobectomy and segmentectomy with radical lymph node dissection. Ann Thorac Surg 2013;96(3):977–82.

46. Tsubota N. An improved method for distinguishing the intersegmental plane of the lung. Surg Today 2000;30(10):963–4.

47. Oizumi H, Kanauchi N, Kato H, et al. Anatomic thoracoscopic pulmonary segmentectomy under 3-dimensional multidetector computed tomography simulation: a report of 52 consecutive cases. J Thorac Cardiovasc Surg 2011;141(3):678–82.

48. Oizumi H, Kato H, Endoh M, et al. Techniques to define segmental anatomy during segmentectomy. Ann Cardiothorac Surg 2014;3(2):170–5.

49. Misaki N, Chang SS, Gotoh M, et al. A novel method for determining adjacent lung segments with infrared thoracoscopy. J Thorac Cardiovasc Surg 2009;138(3):613–8.

50. Misaki N, Chang SS, Igai H, et al. New clinically applicable method for visualizing adjacent lung segments using an infrared thoracoscopy system. J Thorac Cardiovasc Surg 2010;140(4):752–6.

51. Volonte F, Robert JH, Ratib O, et al. A lung segmentectomy performed with 3D reconstruction images available on the operating table with an iPad. Interact Cardiovasc Thorac Surg 2011;12(6):1066–8.

52. Bertolaccini L, Rizzardi G, Terzi A. Single-port video-assisted thoracic surgery resection: the Copernican revolution of a geometrical approach in thoracic surgery? Interact Cardiovasc Thorac Surg 2011;12(3):516.

53. Sihoe AD. Reasons not to perform uniportal VATS lobectomy. J Thorac Dis 2016;8(Suppl 3):S333–43.

54. Wang BY, Liu CY, Hsu PK, et al. Single-incision versus multiple-incision thoracoscopic lobectomy and segmentectomy: a propensity-matched analysis. Ann Surg 2015;261(4):793–9.

55. Gonzalez-Rivas D, Mendez L, Delgado M, et al. Uniportal video-assisted thoracoscopic anatomic segmentectomy. J Thorac Dis 2013;5(Suppl 3):S226–33.

56. Han KN, Kim HK, Choi YH. Uniportal video-assisted thoracoscopic surgical (VATS) segmentectomy with preoperative dual localization: right upper lobe wedge resection and left upper lobe upper division segmentectomy. Ann Cardiothorac Surg 2016;5(2):147–50.

57. Lin Y, Zheng W, Zhu Y, et al. Comparison of treatment outcomes between single-port video-assisted-thoracoscopic anatomic segmentectomy and lobectomy for non-small celllung cancer of early-stage: a retrospective observational study. J Thorac Dis 2016;8(6):1290–6.

58. Perna V, Carvajal AF, Torrecilla JA, et al. Uniportal video-assisted thoracoscopic lobectomy versus other video-assisted thoracoscopic lobectomy techniques: a randomized study. Eur J Cardiothorac Surg 2016;50(3):411–5.

Nonintubated–Awake Anesthesia for Uniportal Video-Assisted Thoracic Surgery Procedures

Hui Zheng, MD, Xue-fei Hu, MD, Ge-ning Jiang, MD,
Jia-an Ding, MD, Yu-ming Zhu, MD*

KEYWORDS

- Nonintubated thoracic surgery • Video-assisted thoracic surgery (VATS) • Awake VATS
- Regional anesthesia

KEY POINTS

- Uniportal video-assisted thoracic surgery (VATS) and nonintubated spontaneous breathing represent a less invasive approach to consider.
- It is becoming an indispensable and fully reliable tool within thoracic surgery programs.
- Although anesthesia for noninutbated VATS is associated with some of the same risks as general anesthesia with endotracheal intubation, noninutbated VATS can be successfully performed in carefully selected patients.

INTRODUCTION

For the conventional idea of video-assisted thoracoscopic surgery (VATS), ventilation control and lung separation and isolation were presumably thought to be vital for the safety and feasibility of the procedure.[1] With the advent of modern imaging and monitoring technology, nonintubated VATS has brought a new possibility of breakthrough to this tenet.

In the recent decade, the concept of nonintubated thoracic surgery has once again gained traction. Within this framework of light or no sedation, supplemental local or regional analgesia, and spontaneous ventilation, a range of techniques and procedures have been described. nonintubated VATS has been intensively researched and reported, which has been advocated to be an attractive alternative to conventional intubated VATS with general anesthesia from several perspectives, such as surgical and anesthetic feasibility and safety,[2–5] perioperative immunology,[6,7] and outcome analysis.[8–10]

This review focuses primarily on nonintubated VATS, and discusses the advantages, indications, anesthetic techniques, and approaches to intraoperative crisis management.

ADVERSE EFFECTS OF INTUBATED GENERAL ANESTHESIA

Mechanical ventilation has a series of potential side effects, such as airway pressure–induced injury, damage caused by lung overdistension, shear stress of repetitive opening, closing of alveoli, and the release of a variety of proinflammatory mediators. Atelectasis in the dependent lung is frequent during one-lung ventilation (OLV) with

Disclosure Statement: The authors have no conflicts of interest to declare.
Department of General Thoracic Surgery, Shanghai Pulmonary Hospital, Tongji University School of Medicine, Zhengmin Road 507, Shanghai 200433, China
* Corresponding author.
E-mail address: ymzhu2005@aliyun.com

muscle paralysis.[11,12] The formation of atelectasis in the nonoperative lung is highly undesirable during OLV because it worsens the already high shunt fraction, increasing the probability of hypoxemia. It can also increase the risk of postoperative pulmonary complications. In the dependent lung, OLV induces ventilation-to-perfusion mismatch, and promotes further inflammatory changes (low V/Q regions increased in the ventilated lung or signs of alveolar damage), suggesting that OLV has more damaging consequences than a period of complete lung collapse and surgical manipulation. Ventilator-related lung injury occurs in about 4% of major lung resections and carries a mortality rate as high as 25%. However, subclinical lung injury leading to minor respiratory impairment is more frequent and related to postoperative complications. Protective ventilation with low tidal volume ventilation, positive end-expiratory pressure, lower Fio_2, lower ventilation pressures, permissive hypercapnia, and recruitment maneuvers are all mandatory in mechanical ventilation in thoracic surgery to minimize lung injury.[13]

High-frequency jet ventilation may be an alternative way of ventilation in thoracic surgery, with lower peak inspiratory pressure and shunt fraction, but it required general anesthesia and orotracheal intubation.[14] Orotracheal and bronchial intubation can also have potential local complications, including throat pain, mucosal ulceration, and laryngeal or tracheal injuries. Tracheobronchial rupture may carry a mortality rate as high as 22%.[15] General anesthesia also has deleterious systemic side effects that do not occur in regional anesthetic techniques in awake patients or those minimally sedated. The deep anesthesia used in thoracic surgery has been related to a higher mortality, morbidity, and cognitive dysfunction postoperatively.[16]

The use of muscle relaxants has been known to produce diaphragmatic dysfunction, particularly in the hemithorax, where the lung is collapsed, thereby producing associated complications as a result of residual muscle block. The intravenous analgesics used during general anesthesia, primarily opioids, are associated with important postoperative complications such as hyperalgesia, vomiting and/or nausea, and ventilatory depression. These effects can reduce the patient's comfort, increase the need for postoperative ,analgesics and prolong the postoperative duration of stay.[17]

ADVANTAGES OF NONINTUBATED VIDEO-ASSISTED THORACIC SURGERY

A potential advantage of noninutbated VATS is avoidance of common complications linked with general anesthesia and endotracheal intubation. Patients receiving general anesthesia with mechanical ventilation have a higher incidence of postoperative nausea and vomiting, pulmonary complications, and residual neuromuscular block.[18–21] During conventional VATS, OLV using a double-lumen endotracheal tube (DLT) or bronchial blocker is required. Many clinicians prefer DLT for VATS, but the "difficult airway" is not uncommon in thoracic surgical patients, rendering a bronchial blocker the preferred option.[22] More recently, improvements in flexible imaging technology and access to video laryngoscopy have allowed anesthesiologists to place a DLT even in patients with complex anatomy.[23–25] However, any approach to airway instrumentation that facilitates lung collapse for thoracic surgery is not benign; both DLT and bronchial blockers have been associated with airway complications, including sore throat, hoarseness, arytenoid dislocation, and rupture,[26–31] as well as the secondary effects of mechanical ventilation on respiratory function. Ultimately, the case can be made that it would be better not to use tracheal intubation at all if possible.

Multiple studies concerning feasibility and/or outcomes related to noninutbated VATS have been reported, and a recent metaanalysis has been published that demonstrates similar results to VATS procedures for indications such as pleural biopsies, wedge resections, decortications, or even lobectomies.[32] However, most reports are relatively small case series or nonrandomized comparisons, and were conducted at single institutions. Furthermore, patient populations, sedation and analgesia techniques, and outcome metrics varied considerably, with few studies including long-term endpoints that were relevant to the anesthetic technique. At present, there are only 4 randomized, controlled trials comparing noninutbated VATS with conventional VATS.[8,33,34] These studies suggest that noninutbated VATS is associated with a shorter hospital duration of stay,[35–38] a finding confirmed by a recent metaanalysis by Tacconi and Pompeo.[32] Medical costs in noninutbated VATS were also reduced relative to VATS, a probable ramification of a shorter duration of hospital stay. Duration of anesthesia, surgical procedure time, and operating room time were also shorter with noninutbated VATS. Moreover, metrics that evaluated satisfaction with anesthesia, need for nursing care, and postoperative oral intake were all improved compared with VATS.

In contrast, differences in morbidity and mortality between noninutbated VATS and VATS are less clear.[3,6] Although there are no data that suggest a difference in short-term or long-term survival, evidence does support that noninutbated VATS has less impact on postoperative defense mechanisms, for example, inflammatory cytokines or lymphocyte response, and blood levels of stress hormones,[7] potentially contributing to a lower incidence of postoperative respiratory complications including pneumonia and acute respiratory distress syndrome.[39]

The largest randomized, controlled trial to date was reported by Liu and colleagues,[34] who included 347 patients randomized to noninutbated VATS with epidural analgesia plus propofol and remifentanil (some patients were managed with a laryngeal mask) or general anesthesia with DLT placement. Combining data from bullae resections, wedge resections, and lobectomies, the investigators found that noninutbated VATS and VATS had similar cardiac complications, and although both groups had a zero incidence of postoperative respiratory failure, composite pulmonary complications (air leak, infection, atelectasis, and bronchospasm) were less frequent in the noninutbated VATS group. Mortality was also zero in both groups. Consistent with the study design, there were epidural-related complications in the noninutbated VATS group (back pain, dizziness, and nausea), and airway complications (hoarseness, sore throat, and coughing) in the conventional group. When subdivided by surgical procedure, only noninutbated VATS patients who underwent bullae surgery experienced a reduction in hospital duration of stay.

INDICATIONS FOR NONINTUBATED VIDEO-ASSISTED THORACIC SURGERY

As noted, nonintubated thoracoscopy under local anesthesia in not a novel concept, even in the "modern" era of DLT. Noninutbated VATS was first reported for diagnostic procedures in 1979,[40] and in 1997 the description of thoracoscopic talc pleurodesis with nitrous oxide anesthesia was published.[41] In 1997, Nezu and colleagues[42] reported results of thoracoscopic wedge resections conducted under local anesthesia with sedation for 34 patients admitted with spontaneous pneumothorax in whom preoperative CT scan allowed for targeted resection of subpleural blebs. In 1998, Mukaida and colleagues[43] presented 4 cases of secondary pneumothorax in high-risk patients with severe emphysema or pulmonary fibrosis performed by VATS with local and epidural anesthesia. In addition, many procedures, including pleural biopsy, decortication, sympathectomy, bullaplasty, lung volume reduction, resection of solitary pulmonary nodules,

metastasectomy, wedge resection, segmentectomy, and lobectomy, have been performed with noninutbated VATS.[5,44–47]

Contraindications to noninutbated VATS include American Society of Anesthesiologists class 4 or greater, body mass index of 30 kg/m^2 or greater, heart disease (eg, ischemia, arrhythmia, or ejection fraction <50), hemodynamic instability, coagulopathy, asthma, and sleep apnea syndrome, where dedicated control of the airway is often preferable when performing a surgical procedure.[48] Instead, noninutbated VATS might be applicable to patients with severe pulmonary comorbidity where general anesthesia with endotracheal intubation may be associated with an increased risk for postoperative ventilator dependency.[49] Although patients with a difficult airway may seem to be ideal candidates for noninutbated VATS owing to the risks associated with general anesthesia and endotracheal intubation, the need for emergent airway access while in the decubitus position is probably a contraindication to noninutbated VATS for most procedures in this subgroup.[50,51] Patients who are pregnant and at risk for teratogenic effects of anesthetic and surgical interventions may also benefit from noninutbated VATS.[52]

ANESTHESIA FOR NONINTUBATED VIDEO-ASSISTED THORACIC SURGERY

A critical anesthetic consideration for all thoracic surgery, including noninutbated VATS, is respiratory management. Many thoracic procedures require OLV, and precise attention to hypoxemia is necessary, which is also true of procedures managed with noninutbated VATS. After the parietal pleura is opened during spontaneous breathing, the lung will collapse with exposure to atmospheric pressure, and OLV will begin. In patients without severe pulmonary comorbidities, a face mask with supplemental oxygen is generally enough to prevent hypoxemia. Hypercapnia may also occur during OLV, but this state of "permissive hypercapnia" is generally well-tolerated.[53] In fact, although partial pressure of arterial carbon dioxide is higher during OLV with noninutbated VATS than general anesthesia, oxygenation is typically equal or better.[54]

Intraoperative pain control is one of the most important factors in maintaining stability during noninutbated VATS. The use of epidural anesthesia should be considered during noninutbated VATS procedures owing to the certainty of effect and ability to regulate level with redosing or continuous infusion. Pompeo and colleagues have performed numerous noninutbated VATS procedures under epidural anesthesia alone.[36] In this series, to obtain somatosensory and motor block at the T1 to T8 level and preserve diaphragmatic respiration, epidural catheter insertion at T4 was recommended with the use of 0.5% ropivacaine and sufentanil 1.66 μg/mL continuously infused. During the noninutbated VATS procedure, sensory levels were evaluated every 5 minutes with a cold test.[33] Repeated bolus injections of 2% lidocaine or 0.50% to 0.75% ropivacaine have also been used. The specific anesthetic agent(s) or administration methods are likely less important than diligence in checking the level of analgesia frequently so that the noninutbated VATS procedure can be performed expeditiously.

In cases where epidural anesthesia is contraindicated, a paravertebral block (PVB), intercostal block, or infiltration are viable alternatives. Piccioni and colleagues[55] described a case of noninutbated VATS with PVB alone. In addition, a 2006 systematic review and metaanalysis on PVB versus epidural anesthesia for thoracotomy by Davies and colleagues[56] demonstrated that postoperative pain control with PVB was equivalent to epidural anesthesia as well as risk for pulmonary complications, urinary retention, and nausea or vomiting. Although evidence from larger noninutbated VATS studies are necessary, preliminary results suggest that PVB might not only be preferable when there is a contraindication to epidural anesthesia, but in select cases may be considered first choice. In this series, although postoperative pain control with intercostal block was inferior to epidural blockade, the efficacy in lung biopsy did not differ significantly.[40] With the assistance of PVB, it is likely possible to perform a variety of single port noninutbated VATS with local infiltration and light sedation.[57,58]

In terms of sedation, Chen and colleagues[2,3,59] described the method of targeting on Ramsay sedation score of 3, at which patients could respond to commands only, with propofol and fentanyl. They also demonstrated a method of maintaining bispectral index of 40 to 60 using target control infusion of propofol and respiratory rate of 12 to 20 with fentanyl,[60,61] where the level of consciousness would be appropriate because of the lack of impaired respiratory or hemodynamic profile.[62] Dexmedetomidine might be a suitable agent for sedation during noninutbated VATS. During procedures other than noninutbated VATS, the superiority in sedation with dexmedetomidine for American Society of Anesthesiologists class 1 or 2 patients was not apparent compared with propofol, and the respiratory profile did not differ.[63,64] However, for patients with chronic obstructive pulmonary disease undergoing lung cancer surgery,

dexmedetomidine during OLV under general anesthesia is associated with improved oxygenation and lung mechanics.[65] The use of dexmedetomidine for patients with severe respiratory dysfunction might be preferable during noninutbated VATS as well.[66]

In noninutbated VATS cases, tachypnea may be caused by hypoxia, insufficient sedation, or poor pain control. If the reason for tachypnea is hypoxia, inspiratory oxygen can be increased as a first maneuver. In the case of insufficient sedation or poor pain control, additional or increased doses of anesthetic agents may be required. If those treatments are not enough to stabilize the patient's hemodynamics, conversion to general anesthesia with endotracheal intubation should be considered. Remifentanil can be useful for the patient who is tachypneic without hypoxia.[67] Infusion or bolus injection at small doses may be enough to decrease respiratory rate, but one should be cautious about the risk for respiratory arrest or opioid-induced rigidity. Intrathoracic vagal block is favorable to inhibit cough during these procedures. Chen and colleagues[3] demonstrated that 2 to 3 mL of 0.25% bupivacaine injected close to the vagus nerve at the level of lower trachea in the right thorax or aortopulmonary window in the left thorax could prevent coughing for 3 hours or more during an noninutbated VATS procedure.

NONINTUBATED UNIPORTAL VIDEO-ASSISTED THORACIC SURGERY

The choice of a single incision technique combined with the avoidance of general anesthesia could minimize even more the invasiveness of the procedure. There are several case reports published showing that noninutbated uniportal wedge resection can be performed in an awake patient. Rocco and colleagues[68] described the awake technique of nodule resection, under mild sedation and giving a single-shot epidural regional anesthesia. Under guidance provided by a bronchoscope, a Fogarty balloon was positioned to occlude the lobar bronchus to facilitate collapse of the targeted parenchyma. Another case report published by the same author includes a young patient operated on for pneumothorax, using a similar technique, and noting that the patient could be discharged on the first postoperative day.[69] Galvez and colleagues[70] describe a case of uniportal awake wedge resection under epidural anesthesia in a patient with a previous contralateral lobectomy with the aim to prevent mechanical ventilation n the remaining lobe in the contralateral side.

These nonintubated major pulmonary resections must only be performed by very experienced uniportal thoracoscopic surgeons, preferably skilled and experienced with complex or advanced cases and bleeding control through uniportal VATS.[71] We consider it very important to reduce the surgical and anesthetic trauma in high-risk patients for general intubated anesthesia, such as elderly patients or those with poor pulmonary function.

When performing a uniportal approach, we can easily apply blockade of the single intercostal space under thoracoscopic view. The importance of avoiding epidural thoracic blockade is obvious: if we are able to control postoperative pain without opioids, it will result in faster recovery and return to daily activities.

Recently, Ambrogi and Mineo[72] compared interstitial biopsies under uniportal VATS with intercostal block versus 3-port VATS technique with epidural. They concluded that uniportal VATS biopsies under intercostal block provide better intraoperative and postoperative outcomes.

CONVERSION TO GENERAL ANESTHESIA AND ENDOTRACHEAL INTUBATION

During noninutbated VATS procedures, conversion to general anesthesia and endotracheal intubation may be necessary with persistent hypoxemia, tachypnea, profound respiratory movement, agitation, poor pain control caused by inadequate analgesia, or in the setting of an underlying respiratory disorder. Technical issues such as the presence of dense adhesions, bleeding, or the need to convert to an open procedure may also require general anesthesia and endotracheal intubation. In the rare case when a patient is hemodynamically unstable, securing the airway with the use of general anesthesia is recommended.

A normal, single-lumen tube is typically recommended for endotracheal intubation at the time of case conversion. The simplest intubation technique available is preferable given that the patient is most often in the decubitus position and it is often not possible to change to supine for airway control. Use of video laryngoscopy or fiberscope might be suitable for expeditious endotracheal intubation in the lateral position compared with direct laryngoscopy.[73] After airway control has been achieved, a bronchial blocker can be used to obtain OLV.

SUMMARY

Anesthesia for noninutbated VATS is associated with some of the same risks as general anesthesia with endotracheal intubation; however, the risk profile of an epidural or PVB is generally lower than general anesthesia. According to the literature and based on our experience, in carefully selected patients, nonintubated VATS for major and minor resections are safe procedures, technically feasible and successfully managed with facial mask, regional anesthesia, and sedation. Patients remain stable intraoperatively, without severe hypoxemia or hypercapnia, coughing, or a decreased mediastinal shift throughout the operation, as well as equivalent short-term outcomes and a lesser hospital duration of stay.

Although the long-term benefits remain unclear, we suggest that it can potentially be an attractive alternative of intubated OLV thoracoscopic surgery, especial for patients with a high risk for intubation. In a modern era of minimally invasive thoracoscopic procedures, adequate training of awake or nonintubated VATS surgery will be essential. Uniportal VATS and nonintubated spontaneous breathing represent a less invasive approach to consider. As surgeon and anesthesiologist comfort with noninutbated VATS increases, this surgical and anesthetic combination is on the fast track to becoming an indispensable and fully reliable tool within thoracic surgery programs.

REFERENCES

1. Pompeo E. Awake thoracic surgery–is it worth the trouble? Semin Thorac Cardiovasc Surg 2012;24: 106–14.
2. Chen KC, Cheng YJ, Hung MH, et al. Nonintubated thoracoscopic lung resection: a 3-year experience with 285 cases in a single institution. J Thorac Dis 2012;4:347–51.
3. Chen JS, Cheng YJ, Hung MH, et al. Nonintubated thoracoscopic lobectomy for lung cancer. Ann Surg 2011;254:1038–43.
4. Tseng YD, Cheng YJ, Hung MH, et al. Nonintubated needlescopic video-assisted thoracic surgery for management of peripheral lung nodules. Ann Thorac Surg 2012;93:1049–54.
5. Pompeo E, Rogliani P, Cristino B, et al. Awake thoracoscopic biopsy of interstitial lung disease. Ann Thorac Surg 2013;95:445–52.
6. Vanni G, Tacconi F, Sellitri F, et al. Impact of awake videothoracoscopic surgery on postoperative lymphocyte responses. Ann Thorac Surg 2010;90: 973–8.
7. Tacconi F, Pompeo E, Sellitri F, et al. Surgical stress hormones response is reduced after awake videothoracoscopy. Interact Cardiovasc Thorac Surg 2010;10:666–71.
8. Pompeo E, Rogliani P, Tacconi F, et al. Randomized comparison of awake nonresectional versus

nonawake resectional lung volume reduction surgery. J Thorac Cardiovasc Surg 2012;143: 47–54. e1.

9. Pompeo E. Awake thoracic surgery–is it worth the trouble? Semin Thorac Cardiovasc Surg 2012;24: 106–14.

10. Kao MC, Lan CH, Huang CJ. Anesthesia for awake video-assisted thoracic surgery. Acta Anaesthesiol Taiwan 2012;50:126–30.

11. Della Rocca G, Coccia C. Acute lung injury in thoracic surgery. Curr Opin Anaesthesiol 2013;26: 40–6.

12. Schilling T, Kozian A, Huth C, et al. The pulmonary immune effects of mechanical ventilation in patients undergoing thoracic surgery. Anesth Analg 2005; 101:957–65.

13. Gothard J. Lung injury after thoracic surgery and one-lung ventilation. Curr Opin Anaesthesiol 2006; 19:5–10.

14. Munoz JF, Ibanez V, Real MI, et al. High-frequency jet ventilation in thoracic surgery. Rev Esp Anestesiol Reanim 1998;45:353–4.

15. Fitzmaurice BG, Brodsky JB. Airway rupture from double-lumen tubes. J Cardiothorac Vasc Anesth 1999;13:322–9.

16. Sessler DI, Sigl JC, Kelley SD, et al. Hospital stay and mortality are increased in patients having a "triple low" of low blood pressure, low bispectral index, and low minimum alveolar concentration of volatile anesthesia. Anesthesiology 2012;116:1195–203.

17. Murphy GS, Szokol JW, Avram MJ, et al. Postoperative residual neuromuscular blockade is associated with impaired clinical recovery. Anesth Analg 2013; 117:133–41.

18. Gan TJ. Risk factors for postoperative nausea and vomiting. Anesth Analg 2006;102:1884–98.

19. Serpa Neto A, Hemmes SN, Barbas CS, et al. Protective versus conventional ventilation for surgery: a systematic review and individual patient data metaanalysis. Anesthesiology 2015;123:66–78.

20. Neto AS, Hemmes SN, Barbas CS, et al. Association between driving pressure and development of postoperative pulmonary complications in patients undergoing mechanical ventilation for general anaesthesia: a meta-analysis of individual patient data. Lancet Respir Med 2016;4:272–80.

21. Murphy GS, Szokol JW, Marymont JH, et al. Residual neuromuscular blockade and critical respiratory events in the postanesthesia care unit. Anesth Analg 2008;107:130–7.

22. Campos JH. Which device should be considered the best for lung isolation: double-lumen endotracheal tube versus bronchial blockers. Curr Opin Anaesthesiol 2007;20:27–31.

23. Poon KH, Liu EH. The airway scope for difficult double-lumen tube intubation. J Clin Anesth 2008; 20:319.

24. Imajo Y, Komasawa N, Minami T. Efficacy of bronchofiberscope double-lumen tracheal tube intubation combined with McGrath Mac for difficult airway. J Clin Anesth 2015;27:362.

25. Yao WL, Wan L, Xu H, et al. A comparison of the McGrath(R) Series 5 videolaryngoscope and Macintosh laryngoscope for double-lumen tracheal tube placement in patients with a good glottic view at direct laryngoscopy. Anaesthesia 2015;70:810–7.

26. Knoll H, Ziegeler S, Schreiber JU, et al. Airway injuries after one-lung ventilation: a comparison between double-lumen tube and endobronchial blocker: a randomized, prospective, controlled trial. Anesthesiology 2006;105:471–7.

27. Zhong T, Wang W, Chen J, et al. Sore throat or hoarse voice with bronchial blockers or double-lumen tubes for lung isolation: a randomised, prospective trial. Anaesth Intensive Care 2009;37: 441–6.

28. Mikuni I, Suzuki A, Takahata O, et al. Arytenoid cartilage dislocation caused by a double-lumen endobronchial tube. Br J Anaesth 2006;96:136–8.

29. Kurihara N, Imai K, Minamiya Y, et al. Hoarseness caused by arytenoid dislocation after surgery for lung cancer. Gen Thorac Cardiovasc Surg 2014; 62:730–3.

30. Ceylan KC, Kaya SO, Samancilar O, et al. Intraoperative management of tracheobronchial rupture after double-lumen tube intubation. Surg Today 2013;43: 757–62.

31. Hartman WR, Brown M, Hannon J. Iatrogenic left main bronchus injury following atraumatic double lumen endotracheal tube placement. Case Rep Anesthesiol 2013;2013:524348.

32. Tacconi F, Pompeo E. Nonintubated video-assisted thoracic surgery: where does evidence stand? J Thorac Dis 2016;8:S364–75.

33. Pompeo E, Dauri M, Awake Thoracic Surgery Research Group. Is there any benefit in using awake anesthesia with thoracic epidural in thoracoscopic talc pleurodesis? J Thorac Cardiovasc Surg 2013; 146:495–7.e1.

34. Liu J, Cui F, Li S, et al. Nonintubated video-assisted thoracoscopic surgery under epidural anesthesia compared with conventional anesthetic option: a randomized control study. Surg Innov 2015;22: 123–30.

35. Pompeo E, Mineo D, Rogliani P, et al. Feasibility and results of awake thoracoscopic resection of solitary pulmonary nodules. Ann Thorac Surg 2004;78: 1761–8.

36. Mineo TC, Pompeo E, Mineo D, et al. Awake nonresectional lung volume reduction surgery. Ann Surg 2006;243:131–6.

37. Pompeo E, Mineo TC. Awake pulmonary metastasectomy. J Thorac Cardiovasc Surg 2007;133: 960–6.

38. Pompeo E, Tacconi F, Mineo TC. Comparative results of nonresectional lung volume reduction performed by awake or nonawake anesthesia. Eur J Cardiothorac Surg 2011;39:e51–8.

39. Noda M, Okada Y, Maeda S, et al. Is there a benefit of awake thoracoscopic surgery in patients with secondary spontaneous pneumothorax? J Thorac Cardiovasc Surg 2012;143:613–6.

40. Oldenburg FA Jr, Newhouse MT. Thoracoscopy. A safe, accurate diagnostic procedure using the rigid thoracoscope and local anesthesia. Chest 1979;75: 45–50.

41. Tschopp JM, Brutsche M, Frey JG. Treatment of complicated spontaneous pneumothorax by simple talc pleurodesis under thoracoscopy and local anaesthesia. Thorax 1997;52:329–32.

42. Nezu K, Kushibe K, Tojo T, et al. Thoracoscopic wedge resection of blebs under local anesthesia with sedation for treatment of a spontaneous pneumothorax. Chest 1997;111:230–5.

43. Mukaida T, Andou A, Date H, et al. Thoracoscopic operation for secondary pneumothorax under local and epidural anesthesia in high-risk patients. Ann Thorac Surg 1998;65:924–6.

44. Chen KC, Cheng YJ, Hung MH, et al. Nonintubated thoracoscopic surgery using regional anesthesia and vagal block and targeted sedation. J Thorac Dis 2014;6:31–6.

45. Hung MH, Hsu HH, Chen KC, et al. Nonintubated thoracoscopic anatomical segmentectomy for lung tumors. Ann Thorac Surg 2013;96:1209–15.

46. Hung MH, Cheng YJ, Hsu HH, et al. Nonintubated uniportal thoracoscopic segmentectomy for lung cancer. J Thorac Cardiovasc Surg 2014;148: e234–5.

47. Gonzalez-Rivas D, Fernandez R, de la Torre M, et al. Single-port thoracoscopic lobectomy in a nonintubated patient: the least invasive procedure for major lung resection? Interact Cardiovasc Thorac Surg 2014;19:552–5.

48. Liu J, Cui F, Pompeo E, et al. The impact of non-intubated versus intubated anaesthesia on early outcomes of video-assisted thoracoscopic anatomical resection in non-small-cell lung cancer: a propensity score matching analysis. Eur J Cardiothorac Surg 2016;50:920–5.

49. Kiss G, Claret A, Desbordes J, et al. Thoracic epidural anaesthesia for awake thoracic surgery in severely dyspnoeic patients excluded from general anaesthesia. Interact Cardiovasc Thorac Surg 2014;19:816–23.

50. Galvez C, Bolufer S, Navarro-Martinez J, et al. Awake uniportal videoassisted thoracoscopic metastasectomy after a nasopharyngeal carcinoma. J Thorac Cardiovasc Surg 2014;147:e24–6.

51. Hung MH, Cheng YJ, Chen JS. Awake thoracoscopic surgery: safety issues in difficult airway and use of thoracic epidural anesthesia. J Thorac Cardiovasc Surg 2014;148:754–5.

52. Onodera K, Noda M, Okada Y, et al. Awake videothoracoscopic surgery for intractable pneumothorax in pregnancy by using a single portal plus puncture. Interact Cardiovasc Thorac Surg 2013;17:438–40.

53. Contreras M, Masterson C, Laffey JG. Permissive hypercapnia: what to remember. Curr Opin Anaesthesiol 2015;28:26–37.

54. Wu CY, Chen JS, Lin YS, et al. Feasibility and safety of nonintubated thoracoscopic lobectomy for geriatric lung cancer patients. Ann Thorac Surg 2013; 95:405–11.

55. Piccioni F, Langer M, Fumagalli L, et al. Thoracic paravertebral anaesthesia for awake videoassisted thoracoscopic surgery daily. Anaesthesia 2010;65:1221–4.

56. Davies RG, Myles PS, Graham JM. A comparison of the analgesic efficacy and side-effects of paravertebral vs epidural blockade for thoracotomy – a systematic review and meta-analysis of randomized trials. Br J Anaesth 2006;96:418–26.

57. Katlic MR. Video-assisted thoracic surgery utilizing local anesthesia and sedation. Eur J Cardiothorac Surg 2006;30:529–32.

58. Katlic MR, Facktor MA. Video-assisted thoracic surgery utilizing local anesthesia and sedation: 384 consecutive cases. Ann Thorac Surg 2010;90: 240–5.

59. Tsai TM, Chen JS. Nonintubated thoracoscopic surgery for pulmonary lesions in both lungs. J Thorac Cardiovasc Surg 2012;144:e95–7.

60. Hung MH, Chan KC, Liu YJ, et al. Nonintubated thoracoscopic lobectomy for lung cancer using epidural anesthesia and intercostal blockade: a retrospective cohort study of 238 cases. Medicine (Baltimore) 2015;94:e727.

61. Hung WT, Hsu HH, Hung MH, et al. Nonintubated uniportal thoracoscopic surgery for resection of lung lesions. J Thorac Dis 2016;8:S242–50.

62. Yang JT, Hung MH, Chen JS, et al. Anesthetic consideration for nonintubated VATS. J Thorac Dis 2014;6:10–3.

63. Shah PJ, Dubey KP, Sahare KK, et al. Intravenous dexmedetomidine versus propofol for intraoperative moderate sedation during spinal anesthesia: a comparative study. J Anaesthesiol Clin Pharmacol 2016;32:245–9.

64. Eberl S, Preckel B, Bergman JJ, et al. Satisfaction and safety using dexmedetomidine or propofol sedation during endoscopic oesophageal procedures: a randomised controlled trial. Eur J Anaesthesiol 2016;33:631–7.

65. Lee SH, Kim N, Lee CY, et al. Effects of dexmedetomidine on oxygenation and lung mechanics in patients with moderate chronic obstructive pulmonary disease undergoing lung cancer surgery: a

randomised double-blinded trial. Eur J Anaesthesiol 2016;33:275–82.

66. Iwata Y, Hamai Y, Koyama T. Anesthetic management of nonintubated videoassisted thoracoscopic surgery using epidural anesthesia and dexmedetomidine in three patients with severe respiratory dysfunction. J Anesth 2016;30:324–7.

67. Inoue K, Moriyama K, Takeda J. Remifentanil for awake thoracoscopic bullectomy. J Cardiothorac Vasc Anesth 2010;24:386–7.

68. Rocco G, Romano V, Accardo R, et al. Awake single-access (uniportal) video-assisted thoracoscopic surgery for peripheral pulmonary nodules in a complete ambulatory setting. Ann Thorac Surg 2010;89: 1625–7.

69. Rocco G, La Rocca A, Martucci N, et al. Awake single-access (uniportal) video-assisted thoracoscopic surgery for spontaneous pneumothorax. J Thorac Cardiovasc Surg 2011;142:944–5.

70. Gonzalez-Rivas D, Paradela M, Fernandez R, et al. Uniportal video-assisted thoracoscopic lobectomy: two years of experience. Ann Thorac Surg 2013; 95:426–32.

71. Gonzalez D, Paradela M, Garcia J, et al. Single-port video-assisted thoracoscopic lobectomy. Interact Cardiovasc Thorac Surg 2011;12:514–5.

72. Ambrogi V, Mineo TC. VATS biopsy for undetermined interstitial lung disease under non-general anesthesia: comparison between uniportal approach under intercostal block vs. three-ports in epidural anesthesia. J Thorac Dis 2014;6:888–95.

73. Bhat R, Sanickop CS, Patil MC, et al. Comparison of Macintosh laryngoscope and C-MAC video laryngoscope for intubation in lateral position. J Anaesthesiol Clin Pharmacol 2015;31:226–9.

Uniportal Video-Assisted Thoracic Surgery Esophagectomy

 CrossMark

Sekhniaidze Dmitrii, MD[a],*, Kononets Pavel, MD, PhD[b]

KEYWORDS

- Uniportal VATS • Single-port VATS • Ivor-Lewis • McKewon • Minimally invasive esophagectomy

KEY POINTS

- Surgery is a crucial option in the treatment of locoregional esophageal cancer.
- Minimally invasive esophagectomy (MIE) has been widely used over the last decade for esophageal cancer; there are some consistent data that this procedure could decrease the incidence of the respiratory complications, decrease the length of hospital stay, and decrease the total blood loss.
- MIE should reproduce the same operation as the standard open esophageal resection following the same oncologic principles and must consist of a radical, complete, R0, en bloc esophagectomy associated with an extended 2-field lymphadenectomy.

INTRODUCTION

Today, surgery is a crucial option in the treatment of locoregional esophageal cancer. Esophagectomy has been one of the most complex procedures associated with high morbidity and mortality. Minimally invasive esophagectomy (MIE) has been widely used over the last decade for esophageal cancer. There are some consistent data that this procedure could decrease the incidence of the respiratory complications, decrease the length of hospital stay, and decrease the total blood loss.[1,2] MIE should reproduce the same operation as the standard open esophageal resection following the same oncologic principles and must consist of a radical, complete, R0, en bloc esophagectomy associated with an extended 2-field lymphadenectomy.

In most publications, MIE is performed through a multiport approach in the thoracic step.[3,4] However, these steps can actually be carried out through only one incision. Hereby the authors present their uniportal esophagectomy.

SURGICAL TECHNIQUE
Preoperative Planning

The indication for an esophagectomy is usually made preoperatively based on computed tomography scan (CT), PET-CT scan, and endoscopy findings.

Endoscopic ultrasound should be performed before the operation.

The extension of the tumor should be carefully ascertained, and histology should be confirmed with biopsy. Suitability for surgery should also be assessed, and pulmonary and cardiac function tests must be performed to predict postoperative complications. Early stage tumors are the ideal cases for MIE.

SURGICAL APPROACH

Three main types of esophagectomies are being used for esophageal cancer: the Ivor-Lewis procedure, the McKeown procedure, and transhiatal esophagectomy.[5] Although the authors do not

[a] Thoracic Surgery Department, Regional Clinic Hospital, Tyumen, Russia; [b] Surgical Oncology Department, Moscow City Cancer Hospital, #62, Moscow, Russia
* Corresponding author.
E-mail address: skirrr@mail.ru

Thorac Surg Clin 27 (2017) 407–415
http://dx.doi.org/10.1016/j.thorsurg.2017.06.009
1547-4127/17/© 2017 Elsevier Inc. All rights reserved.

thoracic.theclinics.com

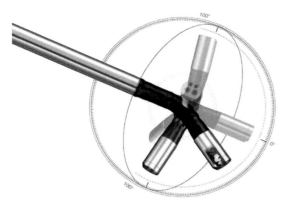

Fig. 1. Flexible full HD laparoscope.

use the transhiatal approach, for tumors located below the carina they tend to use the Ivor-Lewis approach with intrathoracic anastomosis. In this procedure, the first step is laparoscopic, whereas the second thoracic is represented by the uniportal VATS approach.

For tumors located above the carina, the authors use the McKewon approach with a uniportal VATS as first step followed by laparoscopy and, subsequently, the anastomosis in the neck.

SURGICAL PROCEDURE
Abdominal Step

To visualize the surgical field and successfully perform all steps of the procedure, a video system with full high definition (HD), 3-dimensional, or 4K mode is used. Straight optics with a visual field of 30° is most often used. The authors prefer using a flexible endoscope, which allows the visualization of all not-easily-accessible zones in the

subhepatic space and the lower mediastinum (**Fig. 1**). The authors' opinion is that the Thunderbeat system (Olympus, Tokyo, Japan) is more convenient when performing lymph node and small vessel dissection because it allows the use of a harmonic scalpel and bipolar coagulation in a single instrument (**Fig. 2**).

The authors use standard atraumatic instruments for most laparoscopic procedures. When forming a gastric tube, they prefer using a linear electromechanical stapler iDrive (Medtronic, Minneapolis, Minnesota) with the purple Tri-Staple Reload System (Medtronic).

The surgery is performed with patients on their back and with the legs in the flexed position. It is important that the legs are not above the abdominal wall because this position can create difficulties for managing instruments and for the assistant with the camera (**Fig. 3**A). The operating surgeon is working between the patients' legs.

The authors use a 5-port technique. The first 11-mm trocar is inserted either above or below the umbilicus depending on the distance between the umbilicus and the xyphoid process. On the right side, the 12-mm port is inserted approximately in the middle of the distance between the costal arch and the iliac crest. This port is used for liver traction and the introduction of endostaplers during the gastric tube formation step of the surgery. The 5-mm trocar for the assistant is inserted in the same spot. The working 5-mm port for the surgeon's left hand is located on the border of the upper and middle thirds of the distance between the umbilicus and the xyphoid, 5 cm left of the median line. The 11-mm working port for the right hand is located in the middle of the distance between the upper and lower left ports (see **Fig. 3**B).

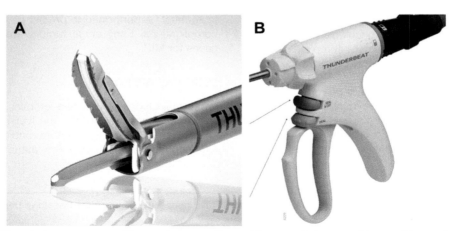

Fig. 2. (A) Thunderbeat system working section curved jaw with a rounded tip provides precision and safe dissection. (B) Ergonomic handle: purple button activates the harmonic scalpel; blue button, bipolar coagulation. (*Image courtesy of* Olympus America Inc.)

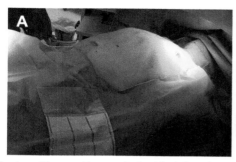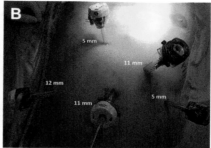

Fig. 3. Patient position on the surgical table (*A*) and port placement for the laparoscopic step (*B*).

Surgery begins with examination of the abdominal cavity because it is crucial to verify the absence of peritoneal dissemination or distant metastases. In this setting, the paragastric lymph nodes are always evaluated.

The liver retractor is inserted through the right trocar to retract the left liver lobe laterally and upward. The dissection of the lesser omentum begins immediately by the gastric wall, along the upper edge of the antrum, 3 to 4 cm to the right of the pylorus.

The peritoneum covering the crus of diaphragm is dissected. The abdominal and intramediastinal segments of the esophagus are exposed. The right and left paracardial lymph nodes are shifted toward the esophagus (**Fig. 4**B).

The next step is the upper abdominal lymph node dissection along the celiac trunk and vena porta. To this purpose, the assistant shifts the stomach downward and to the left. The peritoneum covering the frontal surface of the pancreas is dissected above the common hepatic artery; group 8 lymph nodes are then dissected. One should exercise additional caution when retracting the pancreas with an atraumatic instrument in order to avoid damaging the capsule and minimizing the risk of postoperative pancreatitis. The dissection is continued toward the liver hilum along the proper hepatic artery. At this time, 12a and 12p lymph node groups are dissected leading to the visualization of the anterosuperior part of the portal vein (**Fig. 5**).

Next, the left gastric vessels are sequentially exposed, clipped, and transected. The celiac lymph nodes along with lymph nodes beside the left gastric artery (group 7 and 9) are dissected as well. Note that the left gastric vein can drain into the portal vein as well as the splenic vein, and the confluence can be located in front of or behind the common hepatic and splenic artery. Metal and plastic clips can be used to transect left gastric vessels; 2 clips are placed on the proximal part of the vessels, whereas one clip is placed

on the distal part. The transection can be performed using a harmonic scalpel or scissors (**Fig. 6**).

The remains of the gastropancreatic ligament are then dissected, up to the left crus of the diaphragm. At this point, the stomach is shifted cranially with the assistant exerting traction downward to the colon or greater omentum. The gastrocolic ligament is transected 3 cm from the vascular arcade along the greater curvature of the stomach (**Fig. 7**A). The left gastroepiploic and short gastric vessels are sequentially exposed and transected. The gastric fundus is mobilized and the posterior gastric vessels exposed and clipped (see **Fig. 7**B). An important and useful trick is preserving the omental flap of the gastric fundus to cover the anastomosis in future steps.

After mobilizing the gastric fundus, the right half of the gastrocolic ligament is transected up to the confluence of the right gastroepiploic vessels. One should be extremely careful during gastric traction in order not to damage the right gastroepiploic vein. A completed mobilization is characterized by a mobile pylorus, which, on moderate traction toward the cranial direction, should reach the right crus of the diaphragm.

The next step is forming the gastric tube. The 2 main techniques include the intracorporal (totally laparoscopically) and the extracorporal (with a minilaparotomy below the xyphoid) approaches. As a rule, the authors use the intracorporal technique. The surgeon stands to the right of patients. A lineal endoscopic stapler is inserted through the 12-mm port inserted on the right (for liver traction). It is crucial to place the first staple firing correctly. The surgeon uses his or her left hand to retract the lesser omentum and the lesser curvature while the assistant pulls the stomach downward by the greater curvature (not by the remains of the omentum or the vascular pedicle), so that the axis of the stomach is aligned with the axis of the linear stapler. Typically, 60-mm long cartridges are used to create a 5-cm wide gastric tube. At this point,

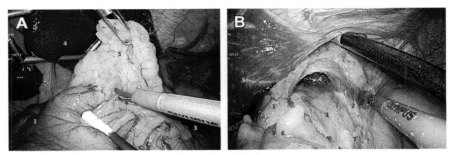

Fig. 4. (A) 1, pylorus; 2, antrum; 3, lesser curvature; 4, left liver lobe; 5, lesser omentum. (B) 1, right crus of diaphragm; 2, left crus of diaphragm; 3, abdominal segment of the esophagus; 4, lower mediastinum; 5, left liver lobe; 6, right paracardial lymph nodes; 7, left paracardial lymph nodes.

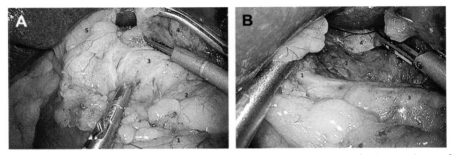

Fig. 5. (A) Lymph node dissection along the common hepatic artery. 1, stomach; 2, anterior surface of the pancreas; 3, common hepatic artery; 4, lymph nodes No. 8 (a + p); 5, hepatoduodenal ligament. (B) Lymph node dissection in the liver hilum. 1, proper hepatic artery; 2, portal vein; 3, common hepatic artery; 4, inferior vena cava; 5, lymph nodes No. 8 + 12 (a + p) with cellular tissue as a single block.

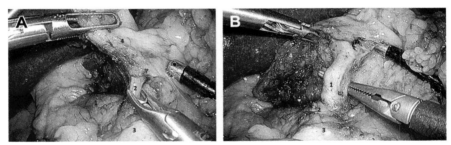

Fig. 6. (A) Exposing the left gastric vein. 1, common hepatic artery; 2, left gastric vein; 3, pancreas; 4, cellular tissue with lymph nodes. (B) Exposing the left gastric artery. 1, left gastric artery; 2, stump of the left gastric vein; 3, pancreas; 4, cellular tissue with lymph nodes; 5, liver.

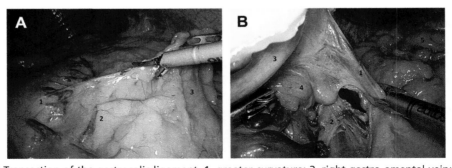

Fig. 7. (A) Transection of the gastrocolic ligament. 1, greater curvature; 2, right gastro-omental vein; 3, greater omentum. (B) 1, posterior gastric vessels; 2, left crux of diaphragm; 3, gastric fundus; 4, part of the omental flap; 5, greater omentum.

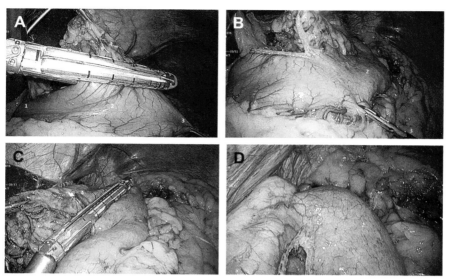

Fig. 8. Intracorporal stages of gastric tube formation. 1, pylorus; 2, stomach; 3, assistant retracting the gastric wall with an instrument; 4, part of stomach removed; 5, gastric wall bridge.

the stomach is not completely separated from the esophagus. The newly created gastric tube is transferred into the posterior mediastinum during the thoracic step (**Fig. 8**).

The final and most difficult step is the wide incision of the diaphragm with mobilization of the retro-pericardial segment of the esophagus and the lower mediastinal lymph node dissection. In order to do so, the surgeon must perform right-sided crurotomy almost up to the wall of the inferior vena cava. This maneuver provides wide access to the posterior mediastinum. The mediastinal pleura of the right lung (and if needed the left lung as well) pleural sacs and the lymph nodes of the right and left pulmonary ligaments are shifted toward the esophagus. The retro-pericardial

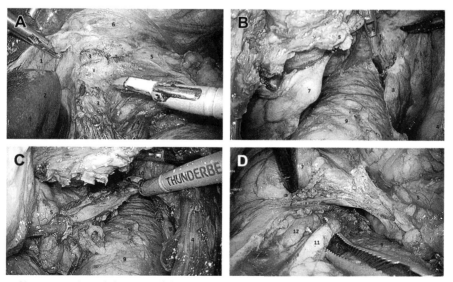

Fig. 9. Steps of laparoscopic mobilization of the lower thoracic esophagus in the mediastinum. (A) Transection of right crus of diaphragm. (B) Mobilization of the posterior semicircle of the esophagus. (C) Removing lymph nodes of the left pulmonary ligament. (D) Thoracic duct mobilization. 1, inferior vena cava; 2, liver segment No. 1; 3, transected right crus of diaphragm; 4, left crus of diaphragm; 5, lower thoracic esophagus; 6, left inferior diaphragm vein; 7, right lung; 8, left lung; 9, thoracic aorta; 10, left lower pulmonary vein; 11, thoracic duct; 12, azygous vein.

segment of the esophagus is the mobilized along with the surrounding tissue and lymph nodes up to the pulmonary veins. The anterior semicircle of the thoracic aorta, posterior wall of the pericardium, both lungs, and the azygous vein are visualized. Sometimes it is possible to mobilize and transect the thoracic duct that makes the thoracoscopic step much easier. To this purpose, a narrow space between the azygous vein and the aortic wall is entered. The duct is then mobilized, clipped, and transected; one drain is inserted in the right subhepatic space to conclude the laparoscopic step of the operation. The main steps of the mediastinal lymph node dissection and the final view of the lower mediastinum at the end of the laparoscopic step are presented in **Fig. 9**.

Thoracic Step

Patients are placed in the left lateral decubitus position. The proper placement of the incision is of crucial importance. Performing the incision at the fifth intercostal space, between posterior and middle axillary lines, helps to adequately approach the esophagus.[6] Using a wound protector is helpful because fatty tissue could interfere with the sutures (**Fig. 10**).

The anterior rotation of the table 45° toward the surgeon facilitates lung displacement necessary to perform the mobilization of the esophagus. When performing anastomosis using uniportal VATS, it is very important to maintain the camera on the posterior part of the incision, operating with both hands below the camera. The authors apply the same principle as when performing an anterior thoracotomy in open surgery, that is, to have a direct view with the surgeon's eyes above his or her hands. Both surgeon and assistant stand in front of patients. After a thorough exploration is completed, the esophageal mobilization begins.

Firstly, the mediastinal pleura is divided posterior and anterior to the esophagus from the diaphragm to the azygos arch (**Fig. 11**).

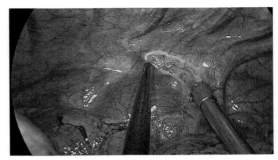

Fig. 11. Mediastinal pleura is divided posterior and anterior to the esophagus from the diaphragm to the azygos arch.

The esophagus is then mobilized by including in the dissection the paraesophageal soft tissue extending to the lung, pericardium, aorta, and opposite pleura. Main landmarks during mobilization of the posterior wall of the esophagus are the azygos vein and the thoracic aorta (**Fig. 12**).

Esophageal arteries are carefully dissected, clipped, and divided. Then the mediastinal pleura above the vena azygos is opened along the spine and vagus nerve. To get a better approach to the esophagus, the azygos vein is clipped and divided (**Fig. 13**).

The authors always perform dissection, clipping, and division of the thoracic duct to prevent a chylothorax (**Fig. 14**).

The pericardium, right vagus nerve, and both bronchi and trachea are landmarks for mobilization of the anterior aspects of the esophagus. One should remove en bloc all periesophageal tissue with a dissection extended to all anatomic structures of the posterior mediastinum. A complete mediastinal lymphadenectomy under the carina, along the right and left main bronchus, along the entire aortic arch and descending aorta, as well as the paraesophageal lymph nodes is performed at this point (**Fig. 15**).

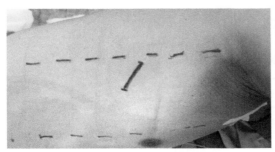

Fig. 10. Patient position on the surgical table and incision planning for the thoracic step.

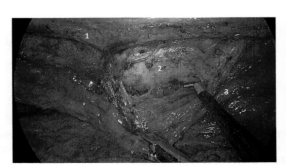

Fig. 12. Mobilization of the posterior esophageal wall. 1, vena azygos; 2, thoracic aorta; 3, thoracic duct.

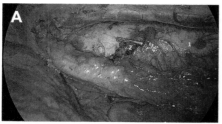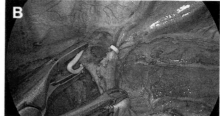

Fig. 13. (*A*) Division of the esophageal artery. 1, thoracic aorta; 2, esophageal artery. (*B*) Division of the azygos vein.

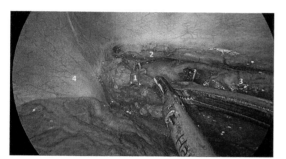

Fig. 14. Division of the thoracic duct. 1, thoracic duct; 2, azygos vein; 3, thoracic aorta; 4, diaphragm.

The dissection of the lymph nodes along the right and left recurrent nerve requires meticulous surgical technique to avoid unwarranted injury (**Fig. 16**).

During the Ivor-Lewis procedure, after the completion of the lymphadenectomy and mobilization, the esophagus is resected with scissors above the arch of the azygos vein. Then the gastric conduit is pulled up into the pleural cavity through the hiatus with the staple line facing toward the surgeon as a landmark for preventing rotation of the conduit.

In the proximal part of the stomach tube, approximately 5 or 6 cm away from the

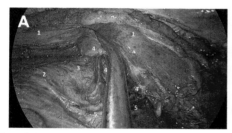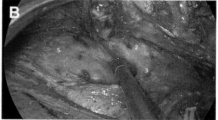

Fig. 15. (*A*) Mobilization of the anterior aspects of the esophagus. 1, esophagus; 2, right inferior pulmonary vein; 3, pericardium; 4, subcarinal lymph nodes; 5, right main bronchus. (*B*) Lump node dissection. 1, subcarinal lymph nodes; 2, left main bronchus; 3, carina; 4, right main bronchus; 5, pericardium.

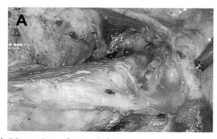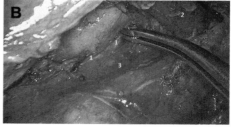

Fig. 16. (*A*) Dissection along right recurrent nerve. 1, esophageal stump; 2, right recurrent nerve; 3, right vagus nerve; 4, right subclavian artery. (*B*) Dissection along left recurrent nerve. 1, left recurrent nerve; 2, esophagus; 3, trachea; 4, left lung.

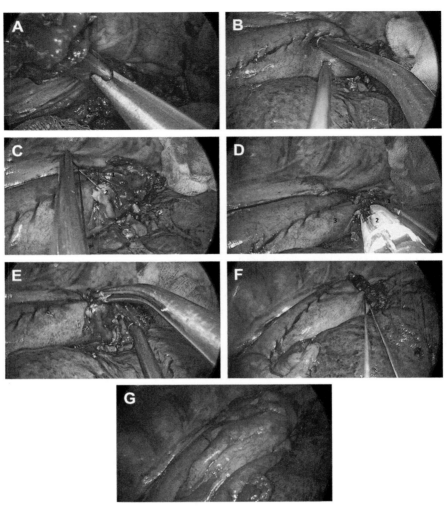

Fig. 17. Esophagogastroanastomosis. (*A*) Resection of the esophagus by scissors. (*B*) Incision in the anterior wall of the stomach. (*C*) Suturing of the esophagus and gastric tube for safe introduction of the linear stapler. 1, esophageal stump; 2, gastric wall. (*D*) Suturing of the posterior wall of anastomosis by endostapler. 1, esophageal stump; 2, endostapler; 3, gastric tube. (*E*) Control of the stapler line. (*F*) Suturing of the remaining defect at anterior part of anastomosis. (*G*) Cover anastomosis of the omentum flap.

top, a 1-cm incision is made. Then 2 stay sutures are placed to transfix all the layers of the esophageal stump wall and gastric wall for safe introduction of the linear stapler.[7] The posterior part of the anastomosis made with the Endo-GIATM with a 60-mm purple cartridge (Medtronic). The nasogastric tube is placed and delivered past the anastomosis by the anesthesiologist. The remaining defect at the anterior part of anastomosis is closed using 3-0 V-LocTM (Medtronic) or interrupted sutures (Vicryl 3/0 [Ethicon, Cincinnati, Ohio]). If it possible, the authors always make cover anastomosis by an omentum flap (**Fig. 17**). At the end, a Blake 24F drainage is placed into the pleural cavity.

Immediate Postoperative Care

Patients are extubated in the intensive care unit as soon as possible. The chest tube is removed on postoperative day 1 or 2. Postoperatively, patients are usually given antibiotics, nutrition, and physiotherapy. A swallow test should be performed to check the anastomosis; if needed, a bronchoscopy is used to clear secretions before patients are discharged home.

SUMMARY

Several minimally invasive approaches for esophagectomy are described, including robot-assisted esophagectomy and hybrid techniques, total transhiatal laparoscopic approach, esophagectomy using right thoracoscopy, combined laparoscopic and right thoracoscopic esophagectomy, and esophageal resection through mediastinoscopy. However, very few publications have focused on the uniportal VATS approach. The authors describe their technique of the MIE using uniportal VATS as the thoracic step.

REFERENCES

1. Biere SS, van Berge Henegouwen MI, Maas KW, et al. Minimally invasive versus open oesophagectomy for patients with oesophageal cancer: a multicentre, open-label, randomised controlled trial. Lancet 2012;379(9829):1887–92.
2. Maas KW, Cuesta MA, van Berge Henegouwen MI, et al. Quality of life and late complications after minimally invasive compared to open esophagectomy: results of a randomized trial. World J Surg 2015;39(8): 1986–93.
3. Luketich JD, Pennathur A, Awais O, et al. Outcomes after minimally invasive esophagectomy: review of over 1000 patients. Ann Surg 2012;256(1): 95–103.
4. Herbella FA, Patti MG. Minimally invasive esophagectomy. World J Gastroenterol 2010;16(30):3811–5.
5. Cuesta MA, van den Broek WT, van der Peet DL, et al. Minimally invasive esophageal resection. Semin Laparosc Surg 2004;11:147–60.
6. Gonzalez-Rivas D, Yang Y, Sekhniaidze D, et al. Uniportal video-assisted thoracoscopic bronchoplastic and carinal sleeve procedures. J Thorac Dis 2016; 8(Suppl 2):S210–22.
7. Irino T, Tsai JA, Ericson J, et al. Thoracoscopic side-to-side esophagogastrostomy by use of linear stapler-a simplified technique facilitating a minimally invasive Ivor-Lewis operation. Langenbecks Arch Surg 2016;401(3):315–22.

Training in Uniportal Video-Assisted Thoracic Surgery

Alberto Sandri, MD[a],
Alan D.L. Sihoe, MBBChir, MA(Cantab), FRCSEd(CTh), FCSHK, FHKAM, FCCP[b],
Michele Salati, MD[c], Diego Gonzalez-Rivas, MD[b],
Alessandro Brunelli, MD[d],*

KEYWORDS

- Uniportal video-assisted thoracoscopic surgery • Pulmonary lobectomy • Training • Simulation
- Education • Minimally invasive thoracic surgery • Lung cancer surgery

KEY POINTS

- Specific training in the uniportal video-assisted thoracic surgery (VATS) approach is crucial to ensure safety and radical treatment.
- A specific VATS uniportal training, including a direct interaction with experienced surgeons in high-volume centers, is crucial and represents an indispensable step (preceptorship).
- Videos published online are commonly used as training material. Most of these published videos are not subject to any scientific control. In this regard, the institution of a specific educational accreditation program for VATS centers to certify their ability to teach this approach seems necessary.
- Technology has allowed the use of different models of simulators for training. The most common model is the use of animal wet laboratory training. Other models, however, have been used most recently, such as the use of human cadavers, virtual reality simulators, and completely artificial models of the human thorax with synthetic lung, vessel, airway, and nodal tissues.
- Another form of training — that usually occurs after preceptorship — is proctorship: an experienced mentor can be invited to a trainee's own center to provide specific on-site tutelage.

INTRODUCTION

The past years have witnessed a huge change in the surgical approach to benign and malignant pathologies of the lung, with thoracic surgeons aiming to obtain the best treatment (in cases of cancer, an oncological radicality treatment) with the least invasive technique.

In this scenario, video-assisted thoracic surgery (VATS) has rapidly spread worldwide and has become the recommended surgical approach for early-stage lung cancer.[1] Its evolution has decreased the number of ports, but in the hands of a skilled and trained surgeon allows safely performing many surgical operations, including pneumothorax treatment[2,3] lobectomy for cancer and other particularly challenging interventions, such as sleeve resections.[4,5] Outcomes of VATS approaches are comparable to the traditional

Disclosures: The authors have no conflicts of interest to disclose.
Funding: No funding.
[a] Department of Thoracic Surgery, European Institute of Oncology, Milan, Italy; [b] Department of Thoracic Surgery, Tongji University Shanghai Pulmonary Hospital, Shanghai, China; [c] Division of Thoracic Surgery, Ospedali Riuniti Ancona, Ancona, Italy; [d] Department of Thoracic Surgery, St James's University Hospital, Bexley Wing, Beckett Street, Leeds LS9 7TF, UK
* Corresponding author.
E-mail address: alexit_2000@yahoo.com

Thorac Surg Clin 27 (2017) 417–423
http://dx.doi.org/10.1016/j.thorsurg.2017.06.010
1547-4127/17/© 2017 Elsevier Inc. All rights reserved.

open surgical one with several benefits, such as decreased postoperative pain due to no rib spreading[6] and reduced tissue damage and immunologic impact, which can be translated to less postoperative morbidity and mortality and decreased in-hospital stays. In cases of lobectomy and lymphadenectomy performed in VATS for lung cancer, results are comparable in terms of oncological radicality to traditional open lobectomy.[7–11]

VIDEO-ASSISTED THORASCOPIC SURGERY IS AN EVOLVING APPROACH

Due to its advantages, the evolution of minimally invasive approaches to surgical lung pathology has led surgeons to decrease the size of the thoracotomy to a few centimeters, through which dissection and division of the anatomic structures and lobe removal are performed, with other ports used for camera, staplers, and lung retraction, according to a center's experience and practice.[4] In this context, the uniportal VATS plays a prominent role, representing the surgical approach to the lung with the least possible trauma.[12] Since 2004, when Rocco and colleagues[13] described for the first time a novel technique to perform pulmonary wedge resections through a single thoracic incision, with the assistance of a 5-mm thoracoscope, uniportal VATS has spread widely; more recently, Gonzalez-Rivas and colleagues[14] have implemented and divulgated this surgical approach to perform standard lobectomy and lymphadenectomy for lung cancer. The uniportal approach has since been extended to more advanced procedures, such as sleeve lobectomy for lung cancer,[5] and in nonintubated and awake patients.[15] Such clinical experience shows that the approach is feasible in expert hands. One of the keys to whether a surgical technique achieves mainstream recognition, however, is whether it can be safely taught to others.[16]

THE UNIPORTAL TECHNIQUE

Uniportal VATS uses a non–rib-spreading small incision (3–4 cm) in the fifth intercostal space through which a 5-mm or 10-mm scope is used coaxially with surgical instruments to perform the surgery.[17,18] For a lobectomy, dissection and section of the anatomic structures, removal of the lobe, and placement of the drain are all performed via the single incision. The surgical technique has been reported for all types of lobectomy and mediastinal lymphadenectomy.[5,14]

The approach to the single-port technique, however, requires a mind-set change in comparison to the 3-portal VATS, resulting in several technical implications.[4,12] Instruments and the camera are used in a parallel manner, mimicking the open surgery procedures. Theoretically, the uniportal approach offers considerable freedom of movement in instrumentation through a single-access point. Bespoke curved surgical instruments additionally increase mobility. In terms of visualization, the direct view of the scope in the same direction as the instruments facilitates the dissection and division of the hilar structures and fissures.[19] It has been theorized that the geometric characteristics of the uniportal VATS are more favorable compared with a 3-port VATS.[20] Nonetheless, technical issues — including adapting to a small single access to perform major surgery and greater distress for an assistant who holds the camera — dictate that proper training is essential for safely practicing the uniportal approach.

TRAINING IN UNIPORTAL VIDEO-ASSISTED THORASCOPIC SURGERY AND OPEN SURGERY EXPERIENCE

It has been debated for years whether prior experience with traditional open thoracic surgery is a prerequisite to embarking on VATS lobectomy.[21]

More recent experience, however, suggests that the learning curve and the capacity to safely perform a VATS lobectomy are not related to a prior experience in open surgery.[22–25] Nevertheless, the results of these articles refer to multiport VATS lobectomies, and to date no such studies have been performed for the uniportal VATS approach. It remains unknown whether, due to the visualization and instrumentation in the same direction as in open surgery, experience and skills in open surgery may be of help to surgeons learning single-incision VATS.

NEED FOR TRAINING IN UNIPORTAL VIDEO-ASSISTED THORASCOPIC SURGERY

Surgeons' independence and self-confidence throughout the surgical procedure should be the aims of training. These can be accomplished with the teaching skills of experienced surgeons, who, through the standardization of training and of the surgical steps, set up the training surgeon and shape the mindset. These steps will pay back in terms of increased procedural safety, fewer intraoperative complications and conversions, shortened operative time, and lower postoperative morbidity/mortality.[26]

In uniportal VATS, the mind-set change and approach requires a specific training from experienced surgeons who explain the technique and the tips and tricks behind it, particularly in the most complex phases of the procedure, such as the dissection and division of the vessels and during lymphadenectomy. Especially in the past, senior surgeons with experience in open procedures managed to shift from open surgery to multiport VATS; in time, they pioneered the VATS multiport approach, standardized the procedures, and then taught other less experienced surgeons/trainees.[7,27–31]

The required technique to safely execute a VATS single-port major lung surgery, however, along with the potential catastrophic events that may occur during the procedure, make a specific training through a direct interaction with experienced surgeons with this approach indispensable.

Unfortunately, whereas VATS multiport technique has been mastered by surgeons in many centers around the globe offering a wide option of training possibilities, uniportal VATS has to date been pioneered by surgeons in few centers This limits the opportunities for direct, interactive and hands-on training — which are central to training because they offer the occasion to interact with skilled surgeons, gain the tips and tricks of the technique, and learn how they manage complications.[32,33] This also limits chances to discuss and interact with other surgeons and even to scrub in during the procedure or participate in wet laboratory surgery.

NEW OPPORTUNITIES FOR TRAINING IN UNIPORTAL VATS

In recognition of the challenges in obtaining training opportunities, there are several strategies for coping.

Video Training

The dramatic impact technology has in life is evident. Technology has shaped ways of living, thinking, and learning. Suffice it to say that connecting devices to a common Internet offers several opportunities for interactive learning, for example, through videos published on Web sites, such as YouTube and CTSNet, where several surgeons publish their surgery and tutorials.[26] A critical aspect of the use of Internet material for educational purposes, however, is that most of the videos published are not subject to peer-reviewed or scientific control. In this regard, the institution of a specific educational accreditation program for VATS centers to certify their experience and ability to teach this procedure seems necessary.

Video recording a surgical procedure (with patient consent) and re-reviewing it with experienced surgeons give an opportunity to trainees to discuss the critical steps and mistakes performed during surgery and to improve technique.[30]

Studies have investigated the potential link between technology and its impact in surgical skills; in particular, the evidence of a correlation between video game playing skills and endoscopic surgical skills has been found.[34]

Simulation Training

Technology offers the chance to train off-theater too, permitting an increase of hours of training to improve and maintain dexterity with standardized experiences, fidelity, and reproducibility in plenty of off-theater surgical hours of training. Different models of simulation for training have been used.

The most common simulation method is through animal wet laboratory training.[35] This provides actual living tissue that allows operating conditions most closely resembling a living human patient. The anatomy is not the same as in humans, however, and 1-lung ventilation for VATS simulation is often suboptimal. Moreover, there are ethical issues involved when sacrificing live animals. Human cadavers are an alternative, offering actual human anatomy. This model is limited, however, by loss of lifelike textures depending on the preservation technique and also the cost and poor availability of human cadavers. Thus far, these models have been the mainstay for training in VATS and uniportal VATS.[36]

More recently, virtual reality simulators have emerged for VATS training.[37] These are excellent in terms of clarity of images, cost, and ethics. Lack of tactile feedback and failure of current models to provide lifelike simulation of tissue handling characteristics still limit their use. To date, a virtual reality model specifically for uniportal VATS training has not yet been developed, but this remains a possibility for the future.

Another interesting recent development is the emergence of completely artificial models of the human thorax with synthetic lung, vessel, airway, and nodal tissues.[38,39] These allow life-sized simulation of operations on human replicas, with the synthetic tissue allowing dissection and division using normal surgical instruments, staplers, and energy devices. The effect is a faithful simulation of human surgery, there are no ethical concerns, and the costs are potentially lower than for animal models. In 2016, these were used for the first time for uniportal VATS training at an international VATS symposium and have shown great potential for highly realistic simulations in future.[40]

Preceptorship in High-volume Centers

The centers, that have pioneered uniportal VATS are fortunately high-volume training centers. These have unique characteristics that allow them to train large numbers of trainees in a short period of time. Foremost among these training centers today is the Shanghai Pulmonary Hospital, which has a fairly legitimate claim as possibly the largest thoracic surgery unit in the world.[41,42] In 2016, more than 10,000 major lung resection operations were performed there. Of these, approximately 80% were performed using VATS and approximately half of those performed using a uniportal approach. This equates on average to 30 to 40 operations on every working day of the year.

With exposure to such volumes, it is possible to offer short-duration, high-volume, clinical immersion training. Traditionally, a clinical attachment in may involves an attachment at a renowned hospital for weeks to months, during which a trainee may hope to see from zero to a few operations each day.[43–45] In a center offering dozens of operations each day, it is possible to see several operations that would only be possible elsewhere after months of attachment. A further benefit of the short attachment duration, thanks to the high daily volumes, is that new trainees can be brought in frequently. Training courses running every approximately 2 months,ensuring that training can reach the most trainees in as time-efficient a manner as possible. Over the past 4 years, more than 230 surgeons and trainees from across Europe, the Americas, Africa, the Middle East, and Asia have come to Shanghai for immersion training in uniportal VATS.

The success of the uniportal courses raises an important concept: that of modular training in thoracic surgery.[42] Traditionally, a trainee would attach to a large unit to learn thoracic surgery in general for many months, with what is learned simply what patients happen to be admitted with in the attachment period. A high-volume center virtually guarantees, however, that patients with a certain pathology or suitable for a certain operation (such as uniportal VATS) present within a short time. It becomes possible for a surgeon to take maybe a couple of weeks off from work and go to a single ultra–high-volume center to learn just one specific item — such as uniportal VATS. Young trainees do not have to take as much time off from work and the trainee's parent unit does not have to cope with one less staff member for as long. For more experienced surgeons, there is the chance to come to China for a short time to learn a specific skill or technique — such as uniportal surgery.

Invited Proctorship

The first steps of training involve seeking out learning opportunities, as described previously: finding material/tutors to learn from and/or traveling to a center for training. This is preceptorship. Another form of training — that usually occurs subsequently — is proctorship. Here, an experienced mentor can be invited to a trainee's own center to provide specific on-site tutelage. Such proctorship has emerged as an important means of training in VATS in recent years.[17,36,46]

Having an experienced proctor come to one's own center has several advantages in terms of learning a surgical skill.[4] First, the entire team of surgeons, assistants, anesthetists, and nurses can all learn at the same time (as opposed to just one surgeon visiting a center during a preceptorship). Second, the proctor can evaluate the equipment, clinical pathway, and other characteristics of the center to see if and how these may need to be adapted to accommodate the new technique. Third, proctors can supervise the early operations by the trainees in their own center using their own setup. This is an especially important step for any trainee hoping to gain experience and confidence in performing the new technique. The proctor may also be able to review videos of the trainee's operations to give in-depth tips and constructive criticism.

TRANSITIONING FROM MULTIPORTAL TO UNIPORTAL

In general, before approaching a VATS lobectomy, experience in other minor VATS procedures to gain confidence with instrumentation (including camera and staplers), angles, orientation, and dexterity is fundamental.[30,31] Also, as discussed previously, the use of the scope and instruments in a parallel fashion mimicking view with open surgery is a good reason why experience in open lung surgery is advisable.

For a surgeon progressing from conventional 3-port VATS to single-incision VATS, a stepwise approach may be adopted.[4,46,47] Uniportal VATS is a product of a gradual evolution of minimally invasive thoracic surgery: from classical 3-port VATS, through needlescopic and 2-port VATS, to eventually uniportal VATS.[4] The gap between a conventional 3-port technique to a uniportal one is big. Progressing stepwise from conventional to needlescopic to 2-port to uniportal VATS, however, makes the acquisition of skills easier. Transitioning from conventional 3-port to a needlescopic approach (one utility incision plus two 2–3 mm ports for instrument and camera), a surgeon learns how to apply the stapler always from the utility incision. Transitioning from a needlescopic to a 2-port approach (one utility incision plus one 2–5 mm camera port), the surgeon than learns how to use right and left hand instruments coaxially via the same utility incision, especially in terms of achieving the required retraction and exposure. Throughout all this, the axis of the operation and the camera views are unchanged, so the surgeon need only focus on learning the instrumentation without having to struggle with a different view. Finally, transitioning from a 2-port to a uniportal approach, a surgeon only needs to become accustomed to viewing the operation from a different perspective — having already acquired the manual skills for bimanual instrumentation through the same incision.

There are proponents of jumping in at the deep end and proceeding immediately from open surgery to uniportal VATS.[48] There is no reason to argue against this when training takes place at expert centers under the tutelage of highly experienced uniportal surgeons. For most surgeons in centers, however, who have not already mastered uniportal VATS, there are reasons why it may be more prudent to use the stepwise approach.[4] First, by moving from 3 ports to needlescopic to 2 ports to uniportal, each increment allows a surgeon to master the component skills one-by-one — making it easier for the surgeon and safer for the patient. Second, if striving to leap too far ahead, the rest of the surgical team (including assistants, anesthetists, and nurses) may not be able to keep up. Should any difficulties or complications occur during surgery, it may prove more difficult to remedy if the team is already struggling to adapt to the new approach. A stepwise evolution again may prove safer in many centers. Third, it should not be forgotten that the evidence for next-generation VATS is not yet mature enough to conclude that any one step is better than another. As surgeons master each step, they may find it not feasible or comfortable to move to the next — and they can feel free to settle at any one step, reassured that there really is no compelling evidence to say the next step is better.[16]

TRAINING STANDARDIZATION AND CREDENTIALING

Among surgeons, the need for reforming the actual trend of VATS courses is strongly felt, because a recognized certified and uniform program of teaching VATS lobectomy is not yet available. Currently, experienced surgeons set up such courses that train several other surgeons without any control over the quality of the course,

teaching, and teacher qualifications. Instead, the authors believe that this is important because VATS is highly technical and complex and, if used by inexperienced surgeon, has the potential to lead to major intraoperative complications. Therefore, the quality of teaching should be high and demanding, especially in the context of its quick spread worldwide and patients' direct request to be operated on with such a surgical approach. For this reason, VATS will become a prerequisite to the new generation of surgeons and, therefore, their training needs. For uniportal VATS it should be no less.

Although the development of common recommendations on training in Europe is a difficult task, a few steps have been moved in this direction; the European guidelines on structure and qualification of thoracic surgery published by the European Society of Thoracic Surgeons[49] outline that trainees should be exposed progressively to increasingly difficult minor resections, that after approximately 100 basic VATS procedures they may be trained to lung VATS major anatomic resections, and that the trainee should be exposed to at least 25 VATS lobectomies per year. This in the view of slowly and progressively increasing the difficulty of the procedure and gaining experience while performing the VATS surgery, ultimately gaining the necessary skill and self-confidence to safely perform major lung resection in VATS. The role of national/European/international organizations should be to act as a certifying bodies, acknowledging those centers that have the experience and the organization to train young thoracic surgeons.

In East Asia, where VATS is better established in many countries, there has been a slightly longer history of credentialing in VATS training.[36,42] This has been done through the Asia Thoracoscopic Surgery Education Program (ATEP), which has standardized a practice of multiport VATS and has certified trainees who have received ATEP official training courses. As in Europe, there is no established certification specifically for uniportal VATS yet — although ATEP has plans to develop this in the near future.

Regardless of the specific form in which credentialing will take place, it is essential to homogenize the practice, standards, and training of uniportal VATS as soon as possible. The over-riding concern is to ensure patient safety, as discussed previously. There is a further important consideration, however. In the early days of conventional multiport VATS, in the 1990s, there was a proliferation of multiple techniques, each claiming to be VATS.[10,21,50] Some of those variations would not be considered VATStoday, but the poorer results reported for them were used to cast a bad light on VATS as a whole — significantly hampering the development of VATS in its early days.[16,21] Such poor quality control over the VATS brand should not be allowed to affect an objective, accurate assessment of uniportal VATS today. For that reason, it is imperative that responsible definition, standardization, and teaching of uniportal VATS must be established.

SUMMARY

The feasibility of uniportal VATS has been demonstrated by multiple studies.[16] Potentially performing VATS lobectomy with less morbidity while upholding the required therapeutic radicality is inspirational to the new generation of thoracic surgeons. As interest in it is rapidly growing worldwide, there is a corresponding need for specific training to responsibly teach this surgical technique. Traditional courses and attachments fundamental to conventional training paradigms may not be enough to cope with demand, and novel strategies, such as interactive learning technologies, modern simulations, high-volume preceptorships, and targeted proctorships, may play important roles in the training for uniportal VATS. Such training may ideally be standardized, governed, and credentialed by national and international surgical societies to ensure patient safety and academic responsibility.

REFERENCES

1. Howington JA, Blum MG, Chang AC, et al. Treatment of stage I and II non-small cell lung cancer: diagnosis and management of lung cancer, 3rd ed: America006E College of Chest Physicians evidence-based clinical practice guidelines. Chest 2013;143(5 Suppl):e278S–313S.

2. Ng CSH, Lee TW, Wan S, et al. Video assisted thoracic surgery in the management of spontaneous pneumothorax: the current status. Postgrad Med J 2006;82(965):179–85.

3. Sihoe AD, Hsin MK, Yu PS. Needlescopic video-assisted thoracic surgery pleurodesis for primary pneumothorax. Multimedia Man Cardiothorac Surg 2014;2014 [pii:mmu012].

4. Sihoe AD. The evolution of minimally invasive thoracic surgery: implications for the practice of uniportal thoracoscopic surgery. J Thorac Dis 2014; 6(S6):S604–17.

5. Gonzalez-Rivas D, Fieira E, Delgado M, et al. Uniportal video-assisted thoracoscopic sleeve lobectomy and other complex resections. J Thorac Dis 2014;6(Suppl 6):S674–81.

6. Cao C, Manganas C, Ang SC, et al. A meta-analysis of unmatched and matched patients comparing video-assisted thoracoscopic lobectomy and conventional open lobectomy. Ann Cardiothorac Surg 2012;1(1):16–23.

7. McKenna RJ Jr, Houck W, Fuller CB. Video-assisted thoracic surgery lobectomy: experience with 1,100 cases. Ann Thorac Surg 2006;81:421–6.

8. Walker WS, Codispoti M, Soon SY, et al. Long-term outcomes following VATS lobectomy for non-small cell bronchogenic carcinoma. Eur J Cardiothorac Surg 2003;23:397–402.

9. McKenna RJ, Wolf RK, Brenner M, et al. Is lobectomy by video-assisted thoracic surgery an adequate cancer operation? Ann Thorac Surg 1998;66:1903–8.

10. Iwasaki A, Shirakusa T, Shiraishi T, et al. Results of video-assisted thoracicurgery for stage I/II non-small cell lung cancer. Eur J Cardiothorac Surg 2004;26:158–64.

11. Roviaro G, Varoli F, Vergani C, et al. Long-term survival after videothoracoscopic lobectomy for stage I lung cancer. Chest 2004;126:725–32.

12. Salati M, Rocco G. The uni-portal video-assisted thoracic surgery: achievements and potentials. J Thorac Dis 2014;6(Suppl 6):S618–22.

13. Rocco G, Martin-Ucar A, Passera E. Uni-portal VATS wedge pulmonary resections. Ann Thorac Surg 2004;77:726–8.

14. Gonzalez-Rivas D, Paradela M, Fernandez R, et al. Uniportal video-assisted thoracoscopic lobectomy: two years of experience. Ann Thorac Surg 2013; 95:426–32.

15. Gonzalez-Rivas D, Bonome C, Fieira E, et al. Non-intubated video-assisted thoracoscopic lung resections: the future of thoracic surgery? Eur J Cardiothorac Surg 2016;49(3):721–31.

16. Sihoe AD. Reasons not to perform uniportal VATS lobectomy. J Thorac Dis 2016;8(Suppl 3):S333–43.

17. Gonzalez-Rivas D. Uniportal video-assisted thoracic surgery. Ann Cardiothorac Surg 2016;5(2):75.

18. Sihoe AD. Uniportal video-assisted thoracoscopic lobectomy. Ann Cardiothorac Surg 2016;5(2):133–44.

19. DE LA Torre M, González-Rivas D, Fernández R, et al. Uniportal VATS lobectomy. Minerva Chir 2016;71(1):46–60.

20. Bertolaccini L, Rocco G, Viti A, et al. Geometrical characteristics of uniportal VATS. J Thorac Dis 2013;5(Suppl 3):S214–6.

21. Sihoe ADL. The evolution of VATS lobectomy. In: Cardoso P, editor. Topics in thoracic surgery. Rijeka (Croatia): Intech; 2011. p. 181–210.

22. Yu WS, Lee CY, Lee S, et al. Trainees can safely learn video-assisted thoracic surgery lobectomy despite limited experience in open lobectomy. Korean J Thorac Cardiovasc Surg 2015;48(2):105–11.

23. Billè A, Okiror L, Harrison-Phipps K, et al. Does previous surgical training impact the learning curve in video-assisted thoracic surgery lobectomy for trainees? Thorac Cardiovasc Surg 2016;64(4):343–7.

24. Konge L, Petersen RH, Hansen HJ, et al. No extensive experience in open procedures is needed to learn lobectomy by video-assisted thoracic surgery. Interact Cardiovasc Thorac Surg 2012;15(6):961–5.

25. Okyere S, Attia R, Toufektzian L, et al. Is the learning curve for video-assisted thoracoscopic lobectomy affected by prior experience in open lobectomy? Interact Cardiovasc Thorac Surg 2015;21(1):108–12.

26. Sandri A, Filosso PL, Lausi PO, et al. VATS lobectomy: the trainee perspective. J Thorac Dis 2016;8(Suppl 4):S427–30.

27. Roviaro G, Rebuffat C, Varoli F, et al. Videoendoscopic pulmonary lobectomy for cancer. Surg Laparosc Endosc 1992;2:244–7.

28. Petersen RH, Hansen HJ. Learning thoracoscopic lobectomy. Eur J Cardiothorac Surg 2010;37:516–20.

29. Hansen HJ, Petersen RH, Christensen M. Videoassisted thoracoscopic surgery (VATS) lobectomy using a standardized anterior approach. Surg Endosc 2011;25:1263–9.

30. Wan IY, Thung KH, Hsin MK, et al. Video-assisted thoracic surgery major lung resection can be safely taught to trainees. Ann Thorac Surg 2008;85(2):416–9.

31. Ferguson J, Walker W. Developing a VATS lobectomy programme–can VATS lobectomy be taught? Eur J Cardiothorac Surg 2006;29(5):806–9.

32. Demmy TL, James TA, Swanson SJ, et al. Troubleshooting video-assisted thoracic surgery lobectomy. Ann Thorac Surg 2005;79(5):1744–52.

33. Hirji SA, Balderson SS, Berry MF, et al. Troubleshooting thoracoscopic anterior mediastinal surgery: lessons learned from thoracoscopic lobectomy. Ann Cardiothorac Surg 2015;4(6):545–9.

34. Schlickum MK, Hedman L, Enochsson L, et al. Systematic video game training in surgical novices improves performance in virtual reality endoscopic surgical simulators: a prospective randomized study. World J Surg 2009;33(11):2360–7.

35. Tedde ML, Brito Filho F, Belmonte Ede A, et al. Video-assisted thoracoscopic surgery in swine: an animal model for thoracoscopic lobectomy training. Interact Cardiovasc Thorac Surg 2015;21(2):224–30.

36. Sihoe ADL. What is VATS? Asia Thoracoscopic Surgery Education Program. 2014. Available at: http://www.myatep.org/. Accessed January 30, 2017.

37. Jensen K, Ringsted C, Hansen HJ, et al. Simulation-based training for thoracoscopic lobectomy: a randomized controlled trial: virtual-reality versus black-box simulation. Surg Endosc 2014;28(6):1821–9.

38. Iwasaki A, Okabayashi K, Shirakusa T. A model to assist training in thoracoscopic surgery. Interact Cardiovasc Thorac Surg 2003;2(4):697–701.

39. Nakada T, Akiba T, Inagaki T, et al. Thoracoscopic anatomical subsegmentectomy of the right S2b + S3 using a 3D printing model with rapid prototyping. Interact Cardiovasc Thorac Surg 2014;19(4):696–8.

40. Wetlab Training Course at Inernational VATS Symposium 2016 London (video). Fasotec. 2016. Available at: https://www.youtube.com/watch?v=D-iEJPftOtw. Accessed January 30, 2017.

41. Zhang X. Current status analysis of development of thoracic surgery in China. Zhongguo Fei Ai Za Zhi 2014;17:518–22 [in Chinese].

42. Sihoe ADL. Opportunities and challenges for thoracic surgery collaborations in China: a commentary. J Thorac Dis 2016;8(Suppl 4):S414–26.

43. Sádaba JR, Loubani M, Salzberg SP, et al. Real life cardio-thoracic surgery training in Europe: facing the facts. Interact Cardiovasc Thorac Surg 2010;11:243–6.

44. Loubani M, Sadaba JR, Myers PO, et al. A European training system in cardiothoracic surgery: is it time? Eur J Cardiothorac Surg 2013;43:352–7.

45. Ilonen IK, McElnay PJ. Research and education in thoracic surgery: the European trainees' perspective. J Thorac Dis 2015;7(S2):S118–21.

46. Gonzalez-Rivas D. VATS lobectomy: surgical evolution from conventional VATS to uniportal approach. ScientificWorldJournal 2012;2012:780842.

47. Gonzalez-Rivas D, Fieira E, Delgado M, et al. Evolving from conventional video-assisted thoracoscopic lobectomy to uniportal: the story behind the evolution. J Thorac Dis 2014;6(S6):S599–603.

48. Guido Guerrero W, Gonzalez-Rivas D, Hernandez Arenas LA, et al. Techniques and difficulties dealing with hilar and interlobar benign lymphadenopathy in uniportal VATS. J Visc Surg 2016;2:23.

49. Brunelli A, Falcoz PE, D'Amico T, et al. European guidelines on structure and qualification of general thoracic surgery. Eur J Cardiothorac Surg 2014;45(5):779–86.

50. Yim APC, Landreneau RJ, Izzat MB, et al. Is video assisted thoracoscopic lobectomy a unified approach? Ann Thorac Surg 1998;66:1155–8.

Fast-Tracking Patients Through the Diagnostic and Therapeutic Pathways of Intrathoracic Conditions

The Role of Uniportal Video-Assisted Thoracic Surgery

Mahmoud Ismail, MD[a],*, Marc Swierzy, MD[a],
Dania Nachira, MD[b], Jens C. Rückert, MD[a]

KEYWORDS

• Fast-track pathway • Uniportal VATS • Thoracic surgery

KEY POINTS

- Fast-tracking patients in surgery has become the standard in many hospitals worldwide; this allows not only for a shorter hospital stay, but also a complete organized pathway for treating patients and improving their quality of life.
- The operative trauma has an important role in the patient's recovery; in this regard, the increasing use of minimally invasive procedures has played a major role in this pathway based on the added advantages resulting from reducing the number and length of incisions.
- In thoracic surgery, video-assisted thoracic surgery (VATS) procedures are aimed at reducing the operative trauma and have been combined with the fast track concept.
- One of the latest developments of VATS is represented by the uniportal approach, which limited the number of incisions to a single 2 to 4 cm incision.
- The main purpose of uniportal VATS is to reduce postoperative pain and morbidity, thereby accelerating the patient's recovery.

INTRODUCTION

Fast-tack surgery is a multidisciplinary care pathway that was initially introduced and applied in visceral surgery by the Danish group of Kehlet in the 1990s.[1] They first described the advantages for patients in shortening hospital stay and decreasing the rate of general complications by accelerating postoperative recovery and improving rehabilitation after surgery.[2–4] Meanwhile, this concept has become a standard pathway in several surgical institutions because of its clinical and economic advantages. This led to a worldwide spread of this system in several surgical disciplines. One of these disciplines has been thoracic

Disclosure: The authors have no conflict of interest to declare.
a Department of Surgery, Competence Center of Thoracic Surgery, Charité - Universitätsmedizin Berlin, Charitéplatz 1, Berlin 10117, Germany; b Department of General Thoracic Surgery, "A.Gemelli" University Hospital, Catholic University of Sacred Heart, Largo Agostino Gemelli 1, Rome 00168, Italy
* Corresponding author. Competence Center for Thoracic Surgery, Chirurgische Klinik, Campus Charité Mitte / Campus Virchow-Klinikum, Charité - Universitätsmedizin Berlin, Charitéplatz 1, Berlin 10117, Germany.
E-mail address: mahmoud.ismail@charite.de

Thorac Surg Clin 27 (2017) 425–430
http://dx.doi.org/10.1016/j.thorsurg.2017.06.011
1547-4127/17/© 2017 Elsevier Inc. All rights reserved.

surgery. Cerfolio initially promoted the fast-track programs beginning in 2001,[5] and later in Europe, Gregor and colleagues[6] showed the feasibility and success of fast-track surgery in thoracic surgery. Indeed, employing intensive perioperative respiratory therapy, thoracic peridural analgesia, forced mobilization, and an early start of postoperative physiotherapy, they decreased the rate of general complications and accelerated the recovery after thoracic surgery. Nowadays, several groups apply this concept in their thoracic surgery centers all over the world.

Video-assisted thoracic surgery (VATS) plays an important role in reducing surgical trauma and shortening the postoperative recovery period. Around 2010, and especially after the introduction of uniportal VATS for major lung resections,[7] this procedure gained more acceptance worldwide. With that technique, the incisions were further reduced to only 1 single small incision so that the surgical trauma is further reduced. The combination of uniportal VATS in the fast-track surgery concept could add advantages in terms of the intraoperative and postoperative part of this pathway.

This article presents a review of the current literature and the authors' pathway in combining uniportal VATS with the fast-track concept in thoracic surgery.

BASIC PRINCIPLES OF THE FAST-TRACK PATHWAY

The fast-track concept in surgery is an interdisciplinary, multimodal perioperative pathway for optimizing the postoperative recovery, reducing general complications and morbidity, and improving patients' quality of life.[8] The strength of fast-track surgery depends on a well-integrated and established pathway that combines preoperative patient training, optimized anesthesia, minimal-invasive surgery and effective postoperative analgesic therapy and rehabilitation.

There are several publications that have been stating the important role of the fast-track system in thoracic surgery during the past decade. In a recent meta-analysis, Xia and colleagues[9] showed how the fast-track pathway safely and effectively accelerates the recovery of patients with lung cancer. It must be pointed out that their conclusions are valid not only for patients undergoing minor pulmonary resections but above all after major lung resections and even for pneumonectomy. In fact, in a randomized trial, Dong and colleagues[10] concluded that fast-track surgery not only accelerates postoperative recovery and reduces hospital stay, but also decreases total medical costs of

patients compared with traditional management. One of the key points in the postoperative care after major lung resections is the management of chest drains. This can lead to a prolonged hospital stay if not correctly managed. However, until now this topic in the fast-track scenario has been a matter of debate. Prospective observational studies[11] and a metanalysis[12] state that chest tube duration is a crucial point in determining postoperative outcomes, and further multicenter studies are needed for evaluating the best timing for drainage removal according to variations of body sizes among different ethnicity. The role of multiportal VATS in fast-track pathways has been also evaluated. A prospective randomized study by Asteriou and colleagues[13] proved that VATS is significantly associated with a shorter duration of hospital stay and increases patients' quality of life.

THE ROLE OF UNIPORTAL VIDEO-ASSISTED THORACIC SURGERY

One of the latest developments of minimally invasive thoracic surgery is uniportal VATS. The advantages of this technique have been already described by Rocco and colleagues[14,15] in several previous publications. Since the first uniportal VATS for major lung resection in 2010,[7] there has been a worldwide spread of this technique.[16–19] The reduction of the number of incisions could lead to the reduction of postoperative pain and morbidity after uniportal VATS. Nowadays, several institutions have changed their technique to uniportal VATS procedures and combine it with their previous experience in the fast-track concept. The combination of the least minimally invasive technique with the well-established fast-track thoracic pathway could lead to an optimized hospital stay and treatment, especially for patients affected by lung cancer.

OWN EXPERIENCE WITH THE FAST-TRACK PATHWAY AND UNIPORTAL VIDEO-ASSISTED THORACIC SURGERY
Preoperative Outpatient Period

The fast-tract pathway could differ between minor and major lung resection surgery and starts with the first contact with the patient (**Box 1**). All the examinations and diagnostics should be performed in the outpatient clinic. In special circumstances, it could be necessary to admit the patient for completing evaluations and diagnostics.

The physiotherapeutic measures can be also started by teaching and training the patient on simple breathing exercises aimed at improving

Box 1
Fast-track thoracic surgery for patients undergoing uniportal video-assisted thoracic surgery

Outpatient procedures
- All examinations (positron emission tomography/computed tomography, cMRI, lung function analysis, bronchoscopy/endobronchial ultrasound)
- General evaluation of the patient
- Patient consent (surgery, anesthesiology)
- Preoperative physiotherapy
- Motivational talks (only 1 small incision, postoperative mobilization, physiotherapy)
- Plan patient admission on operation day

Preoperative/operation day
- Marking the operation side
- Motivational talks
- Oral intake until 4 hours before surgery, drink clear fluids until 2 hours before surgery
- Take own long-term medications

Intraoperative
- Check the identity of the patient
- No central venous catheter
- Comfort positioning of the patient
- Antibiotic prophylaxis (repeat after 2 hours)
- Control room temperature
- Intercostal nerve block at the beginning and end
- No rib spreading
- Use wound protector to prevent tumor seeding
- Extubation of patient in operating room
- Transfer patient to intermediate care unit
- ICU only if necessary

Postoperative operation day
- At the intermediate care unit/ICU
  - Drinking 2 hours after surgery
  - RR and HF control
  - Blood gas analysis
  - No radiograph
  - Control for air leakage
  - Start continuous positive airway pressure
  - Speak to the family
  - Motivational talks
- At the ward
  - 5 hours after the operation stand and walk in the room
  - Sit for 2 hours
  - Eat after 5 hours
  - Pain therapy according to VAS

First postoperative day
- 2x RR + HF control
- Laboratory
- Radiograph
- Check for air leakage
- Motivational talks with patient and family
- Physiotherapy (breathing exercises and walking in the ward)

Second postoperative day
- Pain therapy according to VAS
- No laboratory tests
- If radiographs good, secretion below 400 mL, and no air leakage, then remove drain
- Motivational talks

Third postoperative day
- If laboratory tests and radiographs good, and patient well, then discharge the patient
- Motivational talks with patient and family
- Explanation of the further procedures
- Try to reduce the pain therapy

Eighth postoperative day/outpatient visit
- Control wound and remove any suture
- Stop pain therapy if possible
- Explain histologic findings
- Plan postoperative follow-up/chemotherapy/radiotherapy

lung functionality and clearance of secretions. In this way, the patient can apply these trainings also after the operation. Motivational talks with patients are extremely important; patients must understand that they play an important role in the recovery process. Every time the necessity to be pain-free and completely mobilized must be clarified to the patient by each health care operator. After completing all necessary evaluations, the patient can be admitted on the same day of operation. For special reasons, like elderly patients, patients living far away from the hospital or for patient preference, the admission can be done on the day before the operation.

Preoperative Period

The preoperative period starts upon admission of the patient on the operation day. The patient is allowed to have oral intake till 4 hours prior to surgery and can drink clear fluids until 2 hours before the operation and can take home medications even shortly before the operation. The motivation talks have to take place. The operation side must be controlled and marked.

Intraoperative Period

In the operation room, the patient must be positioned in a relaxed correct position for preventing any lesion due to an incorrect positioning. For this reason, a vacuum mattress can be employed. The patient must be at a right temperature during the operation, using thermal blankets, for achieving early extubation. The antibiotic prophylaxis is given as a single shot before the start of the operation and repeated after 2 hours. Deep venous thrombosis (DVT) prevention devices must be used. The operative trauma is reduced by using the uniportal VATS technique. A small incision is performed in this approach (2–4 cm),[20] preventing muscle disruption and rib spreading. A wound protector is used to prevent cutaneous infections and tumor cell seeding. It is important to choose the right intercostal space to prevent excessive angulation and pressure on the rib by the instruments. The intercostal blockade is performed using ropivacain and repeated at the end of the procedure; it greatly contributes to postoperative analgesia.[20,21] At the end of the procedure, only 1 thoracic drain 24 Ch is placed through the same incision.[20] A digital air leak measurement is preferred. The patient is extubated in the operating room.

Postoperative Period – Operation Day

Patients after major lung resection should be admitted to the intermediate care unit, where they are monitored for 2 to 6 hours. In special circumstances, the patient can be admitted to the intensive care unit (ICU). During this phase, the patient should be monitored and undergo blood examinations and hemogasanalysis. No chest radiograph is necessary on the day of the operation. Chest drainage should be set on a negative pressure of -7 cm H_2O. When the patient is back on the ward, the nurses should measure the blood pressure and the heart rate. The surgeon on duty should check the patient, to evaluate the level of pain and quality and amount of fluid in the drainage. No fluid infusion is necessary on the ward, because 2 hours after the operation the patient can restart oral intake, drinking yoghurt and protein drinks. After 5 hours, the patient can go on a solid diet. Six hours after operation, antithrombotic prophylaxis with low molecular weight heparin (according to the patient's weight) must be administered. Breathing exercises start immediately after the operation. Five hours after operation, the physiotherapy and mobilization of the patient start in the room, keeping the patient sitting for 2 hours in a chair. It is important to speak with the patient to motivate him or her to exercise and to proceed with respiratory training according to the modality already learned before operation.

POSTOPERATIVE PERIOD – FROM THE FIRST POSTOPERATIVE DAY

From the first postoperative day, the patient must be motivated to restore a standard of life closer to that one he or she had before the operation, especially with regard to food and movement. A chest radiograph is performed, and the amount and quality of effusion from chest drainage are evaluated. If the amount is less tan 400 mL and no air leakage is detected, the drainage can be removed 24 to 72 hours after the operation. On the day of chest tube removal, the patient can be also discharged. All patients are reviewed at the outpatient clinic to check the wounds, remove sutures if necessary, and to plan the further therapy or follow-up according to the final pathology.

SUMMARY

The uniportal VATS technique is among the least invasive surgical procedures in thoracic surgery.

Only 1 small incision is performed without any rib spreading, which decreases the surgical trauma. According to the authors' experience, the combination between uniportal VATS and fast-track surgery may provide real and important advantages for the patient in terms of recovery, reduction of postoperative morbidity, and improvement of quality of life. Indeed, an increasing number of publications has already described the effectiveness of the fast-track program in terms of economic advantages and recovery for the patients both for other general thoracic surgical procedures and uniportal VATS operations. Only a few reports, however, evaluate the results of both combined. Further prospective and randomized studies on more sophisticated and up-to-date thoracic fast-track programs, including the ones based on the uniportal VATS technique, are necessary to provide data and define certain conclusions.

REFERENCES

1. Kehlet H. Multimodal approach to control postoperative pathophysiology and rehabilitation. Br J Anaesth 1997;78(5):606–17.
2. Basse L, Hjort Jakobsen D, Billesbolle P, et al. A clinical pathway to accelerate recovery after colonic resection. Ann Surg 2000;232:51–7.
3. Basse L, Raskov HH, Hjort Jakobsen D, et al. Accelerated postoperative recovery programme after colonic resection improves physical performance, pulmonary function and body composition. Br J Surg 2002;89:446–53.
4. Basse L, Thorbol JE, Lossl K, et al. Colonic surgery with accelerated rehabilitation or conventional care. Dis Colon Rectum 2004;47:271–7.
5. Cerfolio RJ, Pickens A, Bass C, et al. Fast-tracking pulmonary resections. J Thorac Cardiovasc Surg 2001;122:318–24.
6. Gregor JI, Schwenk W, Mall J, et al. "Fast-track" rehabilitation in thoracic surgery. First experiences with a multimodal, interdisciplinary, and proven perioperative treatment course. Chirurg 2008;79(7): 657–64.
7. Gonzalez-Rivas D, Paradela M, Fernandez R, et al. Uniportal video-assisted thoracoscopic lobectomy: two years of experience. Ann Thorac Surg 2013; 95(2):426–32.
8. Schwenk W, Müller JM. What is "fast-track"-surgery? Dtsch Med Wochenschr 2005;130(10):536–40.
9. Xia Y, Chang S, Ye J, et al. Application effect of fast track surgery for patients with lung cancer: a meta-analysis. Zhongguo Fei Ai Za Zhi 2016; 19(12):827–36.
10. Dong Q, Zhang K, Cao S, et al. Fast-track surgery versus conventional perioperative management of

lung cancer-associated pneumonectomy: a randomized controlled clinical trial. World J Surg Oncol 2017;15(1):20.

11. Dumans-Nizard V, Guezennec J, Parquin F, et al. Feasibility and results of a fast-track protocol in thoracic surgery. Minerva Anestesiol 2016;82:15–21.

12. Deng B, Qian K, Zhou JH, et al. Optimization of chest tube management to expedite rehabilitation of lung cancer patients after video-assisted thoracic surgery: a meta-analysis and systematic review. World J Surg 2017. http://dx.doi.org/10.1007/s00268-017-3975-x.

13. Asteriou C, Lazopoulos A, Rallis T, et al. Fast-track rehabilitation following video-assisted pulmonary sublobar wedge resection: a prospective randomized study. J Minim Access Surg 2016;12(3):209–13.

14. Rocco G, Martin-Ucar A, Passera E. Uniportal VATS wedge pulmonary resections. Ann Thorac Surg 2004;77(2):726–8.

15. Jutley RS, Khalil MW, Rocco G. Uniportal vs standard three-port VATS technique for spontaneous pneumothorax: comparison of post-operative pain and residual paraesthesia. Eur J Cardiothorac Surg 2005;28(1):43–6.

16. Wang L, Liu D, Lu J, et al. The feasibility and advantage of uniportal video-assisted thoracoscopic surgery (VATS) in pulmonary lobectomy. BMC Cancer 2017;17(1):75.

17. Abu Akar F, Gonzalez-Rivas D, Ismail M, et al. Uniportal video-assisted thoracic surgery: the Middle East experience. J Thorac Dis 2017;9(4):871–7.

18. De Oliveira A, Couto TAPP. The development of uniportal video - assisted thoracoscopic surgery in São Paulo: from diagnosis to lobectomy. J Thorac Dis 2017;9(4):865–70.

19. Bedetti B, Bertolaccini L, Solli P, et al. Learning curve and established phase for uniportal VATS lobectomies: the Papworth experience. J Thorac Dis 2017;9(1):138–42.

20. Ismail M, Swierzy M, Nachira D, et al. Uniportal video-assisted thoracic surgery for major lung resections: pitfalls, tips and tricks. J Thorac Dis 2017;9(4):885–97.

21. Komatsu T, Kino A, Inoue M, et al. Paravertebral block for video-assisted thoracoscopic surgery: analgesic effectiveness and role in fast-track surgery. Int J Surg 2014;12(9):936–9.

UNITED STATES POSTAL SERVICE ® Statement of Ownership, Management, and Circulation (All Periodicals Publications Except Requester Publications)

1. Publication Title	2. Publication Number	3. Filing Date
THORACIC SURGERY CLINICS	013 – 126	9/18/2017

4. Issue Frequency	5. Number of Issues Published Annually	6. Annual Subscription Price
FEB, MAY, AUG, NOV	4	$359.00

7. Complete Mailing Address of Known Office of Publication (Not printer) (Street, city, county, state, and ZIP+4®)

ELSEVIER INC.
230 Park Avenue, Suite 800
New York, NY 10169

Contact Person: STEPHEN R. BUSHING
Telephone (Include area code): 215-239-3688

8. Complete Mailing Address of Headquarters or General Business Office of Publisher (Not printer)

ELSEVIER INC.
230 Park Avenue, Suite 800
New York, NY 10169

9. Full Names and Complete Mailing Addresses of Publisher, Editor, and Managing Editor (Do not leave blank)

Publisher (Name and complete mailing address)

ADRIANNE BRIGIDO, ELSEVIER INC.
1600 JOHN F KENNEDY BLVD. SUITE 1800
PHILADELPHIA, PA 19103-2899

Editor (Name and complete mailing address)

JOHN VASSALLO, ELSEVIER INC.
1600 JOHN F KENNEDY BLVD. SUITE 1800
PHILADELPHIA, PA 19103-2899

Managing Editor (Name and complete mailing address)

PATRICK MANLEY, ELSEVIER INC.
1600 JOHN F KENNEDY BLVD. SUITE 1800
PHILADELPHIA, PA 19103-2899

10. Owner (Do not leave blank. If the publication is owned by a corporation, give the name and address of the corporation immediately followed by the names and addresses of all stockholders owning or holding 1 percent or more of the total amount of stock. If not owned by a corporation, give the names and addresses of the individual owners. If owned by a partnership or other unincorporated firm, give its name and address as well as those of each individual owner. If the publication is published by a nonprofit organization, give its name and address.)

Full Name	Complete Mailing Address
WHOLLY OWNED SUBSIDIARY OF REED/ELSEVIER, US HOLDINGS	1600 JOHN F KENNEDY BLVD. SUITE 1800 PHILADELPHIA, PA 19103-2899

11. Known Bondholders, Mortgagees, and Other Security Holders Owning or Holding 1 Percent or More of Total Amount of Bonds, Mortgages, or Other Securities. If none, check box ▶ ☐ None

Full Name	Complete Mailing Address
N/A	

12. Tax Status (For completion by nonprofit organizations authorized to mail at nonprofit rates) (Check one)
The purpose, function, and nonprofit status of this organization and the exempt status for federal income tax purposes:
☒ Has Not Changed During Preceding 12 Months
☐ Has Changed During Preceding 12 Months (Publisher must submit explanation of change with this statement)

PS Form **3526**, July 2014 (Page 1 of 4 (see instructions page 4)) PSN 7530-01-000-9931 PRIVACY NOTICE: See our privacy policy on www.usps.com.

---

13. Publication Title	14. Issue Date for Circulation Data Below
THORACIC SURGERY CLINICS	AUGUST 2017

15. Extent and Nature of Circulation

		Average No. Copies Each Issue During Preceding 12 Months	No. Copies of Single Issue Published Nearest to Filing Date
a. Total Number of Copies (Net press run)		407	304
b. Paid Circulation (By Mail and Outside the Mail)	(1) Mailed Outside-County Paid Subscriptions Stated on PS Form 3541 (Include paid distribution above nominal rate, advertiser's proof copies, and exchange copies)	167	149
	(2) Mailed In-County Paid Subscriptions Stated on PS Form 3541 (Include paid distribution above nominal rate, advertiser's proof copies, and exchange copies)	0	0
	(3) Paid Distribution Outside the Mails Including Sales Through Dealers and Carriers, Street Vendors, Counter Sales, and Other Paid Distribution Outside USPS®	118	99
	(4) Paid Distribution by Other Classes of Mail Through the USPS (e.g. First-Class Mail®)	0	0
c. Total Paid Distribution (Sum of 15b (1), (2), (3), and (4))	▶	285	248
d. Free or Nominal Rate Distribution (By Mail and Outside the Mail)	(1) Free or Nominal Rate Outside-County Copies included on PS Form 3541	58	56
	(2) Free or Nominal Rate In-County Copies Included on PS Form 3541	0	0
	(3) Free or Nominal Rate Copies Mailed at Other Classes Through the USPS (e.g. First-Class Mail)	0	0
	(4) Free or Nominal Rate Distribution Outside the Mail (Carriers or other means)	0	0
e. Total Free or Nominal Rate Distribution (Sum of 15d (1), (2), (3) and (4))	▶	58	56
f. Total Distribution (Sum of 15c and 15e)	▶	343	304
g. Copies not Distributed (See Instructions to Publishers #4 (page #3))	▶	64	0
h. Total (Sum of 15f and g)	▶	407	304
i. Percent Paid (15c divided by 15f times 100)	▶	83.09%	81.58%

* If you are claiming electronic copies, go to line 16 on page 3. If you are not claiming electronic copies, skip to line 17 on page 3.

16. Electronic Copy Circulation

	Average No. Copies Each Issue During Preceding 12 Months	No. Copies of Single Issue Published Nearest to Filing Date
a. Paid Electronic Copies ▶	0	0
b. Total Paid Print Copies (Line 15c) + Paid Electronic Copies (Line 16a) ▶	285	248
c. Total Print Distribution (Line 15f) + Paid Electronic Copies (Line 16a) ▶	343	304
d. Percent Paid (Both Print & Electronic Copies) (16b divided by 16c × 100) ▶	83.09%	81.58%

☒ I certify that 50% of all my distributed copies (electronic and print) are paid above a nominal price.

17. Publication of Statement of Ownership

☒ If the publication is a general publication, publication of this statement is required. Will be printed ☐ Publication not required.
in the NOVEMBER 2017 issue of this publication.

18. Signature and Title of Editor, Publisher, Business Manager, or Owner

STEPHEN R. BUSHING - INVENTORY DISTRIBUTION CONTROL MANAGER

Stephen R. Bushing Date 9/18/2017

I certify that all information furnished on this form is true and complete. I understand that anyone who furnishes false or misleading information on this form or who omits material or information requested on the form may be subject to criminal sanctions (including fines and imprisonment) and/or civil sanctions (including civil penalties).

Printed and bound by CPI Group (UK) Ltd, Croydon, CR0 4YY

08/05/2025

01864703-0014